Reflections on Authentic Movement

This collection of essays advances the existing literature on Authentic Movement exploring the history, practice and theory of Authentic Movement which integrates the fields of dance, movement and psychotherapy.

Providing a contemporary and new perspective, the book moves beyond the purely therapeutic and spiritual aims of Authentic Movement and opens it up to new applications. The first part of the book introduces the history and practice of Authentic Movement, describing and illustrating origins, forms and specific expert terminology and explaining their rationale. It then develops an in-depth analysis of particular aspects of Authentic Movement from the perspective of an expert practitioner using philosophy, dance history and the lens of art-making. Case studies exemplify how the practices and qualities of Authentic Movement can aid creative, reflective processes in dance, dance therapy as well as in visual art, film making, collaborative projects and ecology. The book emphasises a philosophical and scholarly approach which is rooted in interdisciplinary arts practices and Adler's Discipline of Authentic Movement.

The book offers a solid grounding and guide to Authentic Movement that will be accessible to scholars and students of dance therapy as well as counsellors, dancers, choreographers, psychotherapists and researchers in the arts and humanities and even in the sciences. It establishes her term MoverWitness as an alternative name.

Eila Goldhahn PhD is an independent artist and writer and the author of Reflections on Authentic Movement: Theory, Practice and Arts-Led Research (2022). She studied New Dance at Dartington College of Arts and the Discipline of Authentic Movement with Adler in Italy and Greece and has worked as a university lecturer, supervisor and dance movement psychotherapist. Her projects and films can be accessed via www.sharedhabitat.net.

Routledge Research in Creative Arts and Expressive Therapies

This series provides a forum to discuss the latest research, debates and practice in creative arts and expressive therapies; including arts therapy, dance therapy, dramatherapy and music therapy.

Reflections on Authentic Movement
Theory, Practice and Arts-Led Research
Eila Goldhahn

Reflections on Authentic Movement

Theory, Practice and Arts-Led Research

Eila Goldhahn

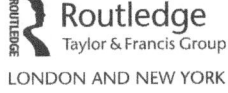

Routledge
Taylor & Francis Group

LONDON AND NEW YORK

First published 2022
by Routledge
4 Park Square, Milton Park, Abingdon, Oxon OX14 4RN

and by Routledge
605 Third Avenue, New York, NY 10158

Routledge is an imprint of the Taylor & Francis Group, an informa business

© 2022 Eila Goldhahn

British Library Cataloguing-in-Publication Data
A catalogue record for this book is available from the British Library

Library of Congress Cataloging-in-Publication Data
A catalog record has been requested for this book

ISBN: 978-1-032-11952-6 (hbk)
ISBN: 978-1-032-11950-2 (pbk)
ISBN: 978-1-003-22230-9 (ebk)

DOI: 10.4324/9781003222309

Typeset in Bembo
by MPS Limited, Dehradun

This is the corrected version of the book that reflects changes made shortly following initial publication when errors were noticed by the Author.

To my teachers and students

Contents

Figures

Acknowledgements

Thank you Wendy Elliott for introducing me to Authentic Movement with your unique lightness and friendship. Thank you for sharing your personal experiences of The Mary Whitehouse Institute and where it all began.

Thank you Janet Adler for being a teacher extraordinaire and an inspiring and wise witness. Your clear presence towards me and my peer group in Italy and Greece year after year has enduringly enriched my life. It has inspired my dedication to the *Discipline of Authentic Movement* (Adler 2002).

Thank you to all the women of La Luna, who together with me, attended those precious years and continue to develop the work in the many ways that you do. Thank you Joan Chodorow for your perspective on Authentic Movement. I feel honoured to have worked with you. Thank you Tina Stromsted for being there in the initial years of Adler's group in Italy and for being my sensitive and empathetic witness.

Without any of you, this book could not have been written.

Thank you Lynn Crane for being my mover and witness during my time at Staverton and for participating in my *Slapton beach movers* films. Thank you Helen Payne for being a supportive friend of my practice and research ever since we met at Janet Adler's retreats in Italy. Thank you for our peer work together and for seeing me digitally during the Corona pandemic. Your constructive comments on this book have been invaluable. Thank you Marcia Plevin for your friendship and for giving me the generous opportunity to teach and film the delightful group of women on Pettu in Finland. Thank you also for the many valuable conversations about the Discipline of Authentic Movement, dance, art and science. Thank you Jaqueline Mayer-Ostrow for being my valued witness and mover during my years in Frankfurt. You deepened and grounded my practice in those years.

Thank you Edward Cowie for reflecting on my questions about Authentic Movement and supporting my arts-led PhD research. Thank you for encouraging my writing and my visual art-making. Thank you Malaika Sarco-Thomas for being a generous collaborator when exploring my initial ideas around Authentic Movement, digital filming, improvisation and performance. Thank you Alan Kirby for being my student and contributor to my research and films. I value your humour and wisdom. Thank you to all the different movers who have participated in my projects over the years.

Thank you to my Authentic Movement students in Devon and London, in Finland, Germany, Greece and Sweden. Without your presence, liveness and your questions urging me on this book would not be. I learned so much from working with you.

Thank you Soili Hämäläinen and Leena Rouhinanen for making me feel very welcome in Helsinki at the Theatre Research Institute of the University of Arts. Thank you for being equal authors to our joint chapter on Collaborative Choreography (Chapter 10).

Thank you, Roberta Mock and Ruth Way for welcoming and supporting my research at Plymouth University during my fellowship and teaching there.

Thank you to my unknown reviewers and Emilie Coin at Routledge. Thank you Amber Burrow-Goldhahn for your reading and excellent suggestions.

Thank you Lydia Corbett for your friendship and the lovely drawings (Illustrations are 1.1, 2.1 and 3.1) of the MoverWitness that lend a welcome light touch to my book.

Thank you Lorenzo Hemmer for your inspiring artwork at Venice Bienale (2009) and to Stuart Young for the photo of me dancing in Lorenzo's installation (Illustration 11.1). Thank you for preparing my images for publication and for your valued support and love throughout this book project.

Part I

Coming to Authentic Movement

Chapter 1

An introduction to Authentic Movement

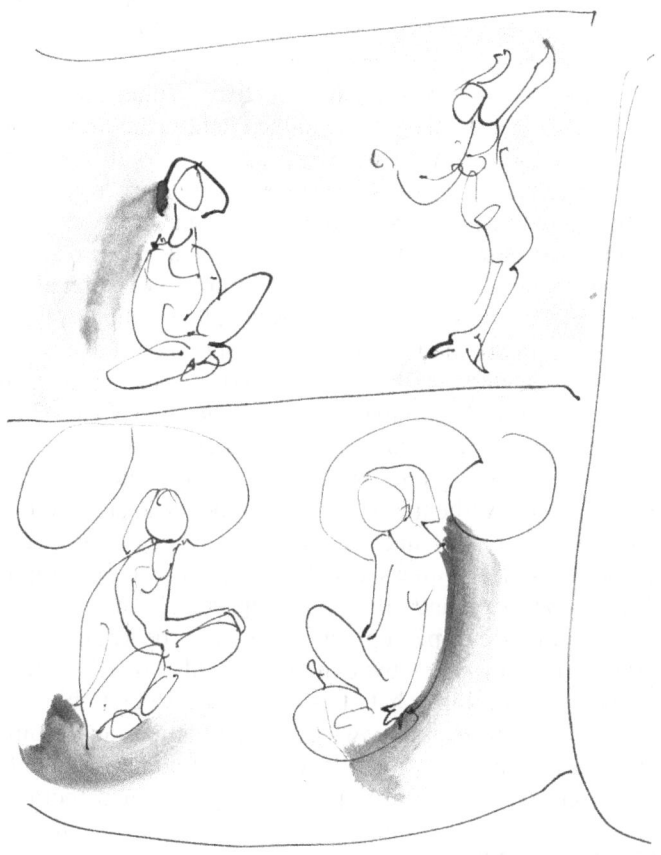

Figure 1.1 *The MoverWitness: the ground form, two ink drawings.*
Artist: Lydia Corbett, 2010.

DOI: 10.4324/9781003222309-2

Introduction to Reflections on Authentic Movement

A person moves with her eyes closed and is observed by another person, a witness. The mover is free to follow her inner impulses in a self-directed way, whilst the witness holds still and silently bears witness to this 'authentic' movement. A subsequent, formalised dialogue between the two delivers the moved and the seen to verbal consciousness. This is the ground form in Authentic Movement. Its elegant framework holds embodied expressions and verbal recall within an atmosphere of warm acceptance.

Participants explore their inner worlds through gesture and movement, and experience being seen in this without judgement. Further, Authentic Movement's particular way of using language allocates participants' unique experiences to the self-agency of each individual. This combination of movement and language, as first comprehensively described by Janet Adler (2002) in *Offering from the Conscious Body, The Discipline of Authentic Movement*, provides unifying experiences of body and psyche, seeing and being seen, non-verbal and verbal, I and Thou and individual and collective. Within dance therapy the witness's role is taken by the therapist and the client is the mover. Fundamentally though, movers and witnesses can be equal players in Authentic Movement and, after a learning process, their complementary roles can become interchangeable. This takes place within one-to-one peer exchanges, peer groups, training and retreats. Authentic Movement networks continue to grow, encompassing international and intercultural, now digital, exchanges of dancers, dance therapists and other movement and therapy practitioners. Since the late 1970s, the ground form and its permutations have been practised in Europe, Russia, Scandinavia, the UK and the USA and, since around 2000, they have spread to Australia, China, South America and South-East Asia. As Authentic Movement practices have evaded trademarking or patenting, they have evolved in different ways according to context, culture and lineage.

The ground form of Authentic Movement appears so simple that it seems to require no particular skill and therefore many deviations on the basic theme of a mover and a witness can be found. Inevitably appropriations have led to some confusion and dilution as important, non-tangible elements, for example a specific use of percept language, are little known or simply left out. Such omissions can weaken the benefits of Authentic Movement and can leave newcomers wondering what it is all about. Regrettably, when used without due circumspection and knowledge, the practice can become psychologically challenging and even evoke dormant trauma. Authentic Movement's psychologically beneficial application by a trained therapist/teacher has been documented by various proponents such as Chodorow (1991), Adler (2002), Payne (2003), Stromsted (2007a) and within topical collections of essays in Pallaro (ed. 1999) and Pallaro (ed. 2007).

Part I Coming to Authentic Movement provides three complementary perspectives: contextual, autobiographical and practical. This chapter traces

Authentic Movement's roots in psychology and explores its shared development with neighbouring disciplines, particularly dance and somatics in the USA. This contextual chronology brings up questions (addressed in subsequent parts of this volume) relevant to a wider discourse on Authentic Movement within anthropology, dance education, performance, phenomenology, visual arts and critical studies. In Chapter 2 A Personal Narrative I provide insights into my own background, exemplifing a Coming to Authentic Movement that is largely subjective. It includes memories and entries from study diaries, encompassing unique experiences of expressionist theatre-making in Berlin and Poland, post-modern dance at Dartington in the UK, and studies in the Discipline of Authentic Movement with Adler during the 1990s. These two chronologies are followed by Chapter 3 A Guide to Practice, a glossary of Authentic Movement's terminology. Based on my trainings with Adler and her primer *Offering from the Conscious Body, The Discipline of Authentic Movement* (2002), it also draws on other practitioners' work (Pallaro 1999 & 2007) and my own (Goldhahn 2007, 2009a, 2010a, 2015). In the Guide to Practice I have transposed key terms and practice elements into pragmatic descriptions whilst explaining their tenet and rationale. Readers discover how each practice element builds incrementally on another. The guide is intended as a key reference point, which readers may want to refer back to as they read later chapters in this book.

Part II Visualising Movers and Witnesses describes aspects of my arts-led research; it explores reflections on Authentic Movement as visualisations in public contexts. Part III What is Authentic? critiques the colonial and modernist concept of 'authenticity' and proposes an alternative term, MoverWitness, sourced in phenomenology. Part IV asks how MoverWitness practices can be applied within a post-professional era to new and interdisciplinary fields.

Note, the term Authentic Movement is used in some chapters to ease the flow of reading. The reader is reminded that the practices referred to throughout this volume are rooted in Adler's personal and written teachings of the Discipline of Authentic Movement, reframed by the author as the MoverWitness. Some of the ideas and essays in this volume have been previously published or presented; therefore, some overlap in content between chapters may be apparent.

Art, the unconscious and Authentic Movement

Early 20th century modernism placed high value on individuality, and artists of all disciplines searched for self-sourced motives to inspire their art. In order to achieve 'authenticity' dream recall, free association and other psychoanalytic techniques such as hypnosis were adopted in the Surrealist art movement by visual artists such as Salvador Dali, Joan Miró and Jean Arp. In pursuit of this, artists looked to their own dreamscapes and found inspiration in children's art and so-called 'primitive' and 'psychotic' art. This development was fuelled by Sigmund Freud's naming of the unconscious. Later, Carl Gustav Jung's understanding of psyche's collective unconscious provided additional interest to artists. Freud's technique of free association to access the individual unconscious preceded Jung's technique of active imagination. Freud's psychoanalysis can render analysands physically supine, in a passive, seemingly unconscious state. Jung's approach to engage deep imagination is a more active pursuit of a dream-like state of consciousness. He placed greater emphasis on a client's own insight than on an analyst's interpretation. In Jungian terms, psychotherapy is a creative act and creativity is considered a source of healing for a client's inner and outer life. In active imagination the client relaxes conscious control of her body and mind allowing images, sensations and thoughts to arise in a dream-like yet awake state in a form of day-dreaming. Many creative activities such as writing, narration, drawing, painting, clay modelling, sand play, movement and dance can be used as outlets for active imagination, also without the presence of a therapist. Authentic Movement too is rooted in Jung's concept of active imagination but it requires the presence of another: a witness.

Psychiatrists such as Jung studied and valued their patients' art and dreams in the belief that the conveyance of images and symbols could assist diagnosis and treatment. Psychiatrist and art historian Hans Prinzhorn went further than this and established a collection of his patients' visual art works. Refusing an interpretation of these works solely in terms of psychology, he promoted a public appreciation of their intrinsic, artistic value. At a time when psychological ill-health unavoidably led to social stigma and preceding the appreciation of 'outsider art', he helped to build a more respectful perspective on clients' personhood and ability, recognising that art works by untrained makers can be accomplished and beautiful. This also applies to dance and movement, and non-dancers can shape exquisite movement moments in dance therapy and in Authentic Movement: no training in dance is needed for a person to express herself creatively using her body.

> Because a phenomenal relationship exists between truth and beauty, as the witness opens towards her own truth she can find it to be inextricably bound to her own experience of aesthetics. While concentrating on the mover's work, especially when a mover is visibly focused inward, the witness can be seized or soothed, awed or changed by a sudden awareness of the incomprehensible presence, the force of beauty itself.
>
> (Adler 2002, p. 63)

In Authentic Movement aesthetically poignant moments can arise undevised and spontaneously, adding meaning to both movers' and witnesses' experiences. At times akin to performances of physical theatre or dance, such special moments occur by way of participants' focused presence.

Such experiences initially guided my questions regarding the connection between Authentic Movement and visuality and prompted my use of film with Authentic Movement in arts-led research.

Authentic Movement's roots in dance

The lineage of Authentic Movement's innovative work begins in the 1950s with American dance teacher and Jungian analysand Mary Starks Whitehouse. Influenced by Mary Wigman's expressionist dance, that sourced dance from within, Starks Whitehouse developed her own way of working; not for performance but for self-reflection and self-knowledge. Wigman, who had created her dances in silence, applied music as an adjunct to her finished works, whereas Starks Whitehouse used movement without music to evoke active imagination. Starks Whitehouse encouraged her students to find their own dance in moving with their eyes closed and described her new work as 'movement in depth'. The inspired atmosphere created by Starks Whitehouse became a key element in her facilitation of movement expression and drew students from all over the USA.

> The studio environment provided an unusually quiet, clean, clear space. There was little socialising. As each person entered, they would find a space in the room, lie on the floor, close their eyes, and wait- or begin to warm-up on their own. Mary Whitehouse was developing an approach that was based on Jung's active imagination. Sometimes called "Authentic Movement" or "Movement-in-Depth", it involved a process of deep inner listening toward expressive movement that was spontaneous – unplanned.
> (Chodorow 1991, p. 24)

Meanwhile, other American dancers granted themselves new freedoms in movement by rejecting traditional dance techniques and choreographic styles. Members of the Judson Dance Theatre introduced everyday, pedestrian and idiosyncratic gestures and movements into dance and sought different ways to perform their new works. They coined an emerging post-modern dance or New Dance, as described in detail by Sally Banes in *Democracy's Body* (Banes 1993). Instead of dancing narratives or emotions, post-modern dance acquired a different, more cerebral flavour and its performances were characterised by abstract, absurd and/or conceptual scores and sets. Some dance became completely devoid of emotion and focused on bodily sensations, movement dynamics and patterns of movement instead. Merce Cunningham excelled in developing this new aesthetic in complex, non-narrative choreographies. His scores, with a wide movement and gestural range, challenged existing preconceptions of what dance could be. His new freedom functioned within clearly set frameworks focusing on space, pattern and time. Music, mostly composed by his collaborator John Cage, was added to the finished works, to different effect than in Wigman's dances. Instead of conveying emotion or drama through dance and music, Cunningham saw movement itself as dance's foremost and complete language. Whilst movement is entirely un-choreographed in Authentic Movement, the concept of movement as its own complete language is a shared understanding.

Almost simultaneously in the USA, where dance underwent momentous changes, somatic movement techniques such as Skinner Releasing Technique™ and Body Mind Centering® emerged. Skinner Releasing Technique™ was developed by Joan Skinner, a dancer with both the Martha Graham Company and the Merce Cunningham Dance Company (Skinner 2004). Body Mind Centering® was created by Bonnie Bainbridge Cohen, who also had trained in dance and worked as a dance teacher (Bainbridge Cohen 2005). Instead of active, creative imagination, as used in Starks Whitehouse's movement in depth, these somatic approaches use anatomy to educate movers. Both Skinner's and Bainbridge Cohen's work engages the imagination and thinking by using anatomical and developmental information together with visualisations. This is different from the imagination in movement used by Starks Whitehouse and her students; the inward focus in Authentic Movement sources itself entirely from within the unique experience of the mover, as she finds herself in a particular moment. However, a meditation-like focus characterises both somatics and Authentic Movement, and that is why they can seem to be similar when, actually, they are different in concept and design. In somatics, soma (ancient Greek for 'body') in all its intricate anatomical, physiological facets, takes centre stage, whereas in Authentic Movement a completely open, non-directive attention takes place. The latter includes all levels of experience and imagination as they arise of their own accord and without prompting. Notwithstanding this difference, somatic techniques can provide valuable preparations for coming to Authentic Movement. From the 1960s, post-modern dancers, for example Mary O'Donnel-Fulkerson and Steve Paxton, integrated somatic work into creative, imaginative processes for dance. Questions regarding such interrelationships between somatic techniques, dance and Authentic Movement are explored in Chapters 2 and 9.

Contact Improvisation also developed around this time, near Northampton University and The Crew House at Smith College in Hampshire, Massachusetts where Adler lived and worked (Adler 1995). Contact Improvisation, created by Lisa Nelson, Paxton and Nancy Starks Smith, together with others, is sometimes described as a somatic technique, but is in fact a form of partnered dance that is used in sessional work, so-called 'jams', and in performance. Contact Improvisation uses gravity and centrifugal force enabling dynamics that an individual dancer cannot experience by herself. By sharing a continuous focus point of physical contact and weight, activities such as balancing, carrying, lifting, rolling, rising, sinking and swivelling become immensely enjoyable, multiplying dancers' potential movement experiences.

Further, the practice of Contact Improvisation embodies collaboration, inter-dependency and trust like no other dance form and these qualities are similarly inherent in Authentic Movement, where mover and witness depend and rely upon one another.

Read within the socio-cultural context of the 1960s and 1970s, all these new techniques signify a desire to supersede the authority of a choreograper and strict dance techniques, and to support performers' longing for greater self-agency and a more 'natural' movement range. Whilst post-modern dance and its new practices broke with some hierarchical structures, they also arguably gave rise to new regimes, such as Cunningham's dance technique and choreographies. With the emergence of post-modern dance a further field of tension was created between approaches from 'within' and approaches from 'without': some where anatomical images and physical laws such as gravity and centrifugal force, as in Contact Improvisation, are used to get to know the body's sensations and to increase agility and strength, and another where uniquely all feelings, images, intuitions and sensations and their expressions are encouraged, as in Authentic Movement. The time when these neighbouring methods arose carried a great promise of liberation for dance. Some of this liberation was realised whilst some of it was stifled in time. Perhaps, if Authentic Movement had aligned itself more closely to the art form of dance, it might have 'freed' and democratised dance more thoroughly and lastingly than post-modern dance and somatic techniques were able to achieve in the long term. But, instead of investing in a collaborative, liberating trajectory within the art form of dance, Authentic Movement's proponents took a different route and became primarily dedicated to developing the new practice's role in therapy and mystical quests.

During the 1990s, Adler became Authentic Movement's most well-known proponent in Europe. Adler, like Joan Chodorow, had encountered Starks Whitehouse's work. Whilst Chodorow continued on a Jungian informed, dance therapeutic trajectory, further developed by Tina Stromsted, Adler interwove her learning of Starks Whitehouse's movement in depth with non-Jungian, humanistic elements. Adler created a ritualised practice, The Discipline of Authentic Movement, a mystical discipline. Perhaps Adler's decision to focus on this direction, and her introduction of the term 'discipline', signified a departure from the art form of dance.

> Obviously I chose the word discipline, but there is still some sadness, because at least in my own experience the discipline is profoundly a creative process because it is based on that which is unseen, unmanifested, not yet visible.
>
> (Adler 2019, video rec.1 hr 19 min)

Adler braided John and Joan Weir's method of percept language (Weir 1975) into her own unique practice. Adler is one of only a handful of authors and practitioners who have acknowledged the use of Weir's valuable invention for peaceful human verbal communications. Weir's contribution to the human potential movement has gone largely unacknowledged. Chapter 3 of this volume describes percept language in some detail.

Adler first described the performative relationship between a mover and a witness and the way in which experiences of moving and seeing closely inter-link. By way of publication of Adler's 1987 essay "Who is the Witness?" in New Dance magazine *Contact Quarterly,* the journal's editors acknowledged the practice's connection to dance. *Contact Quarterly* supported the develop-ment of post-modern dance in general and Contact Improvisation, Authentic Movement, Body Mind Centering® and other approaches to movement in par-ticular. Whilst in the following years Adler's discipline began to align itself more and more with the fields of meditation, mysticism and self-reflection, rather than with dance, an undercurrent of Authentic Movement as a performa-tive art form lingered on. Andrea Olsen, also in *Contact Quarterly,* wrote: "The relationship between the mover and the witness parallels that of performer and audience" (Olsen 1993, p. 49) and "Authentic Movement also exists as perfor-mance" (Olsen 1993, p. 51). She stated that the practice of Authentic Move-ment can also inform the actual viewing of performances (Olsen 1993). Being seen and being heard are the premise of performance and in Authentic Movement participants create confidential, private 'performances'. However, in the fields of therapy and wellbeing, the term performance is often mistakenly associated with a notion of pretence and superficiality. This is a notion that, like the term 'authentic' within the field of performance, can prevent a helpful exchange between these disciplines. Dancer and choreographer Olsen observed how Authentic Movement can reveal dancers' emotional states, par-ticularly fear when being aware of being seen:

> As we begin Authentic Movement we may face basic fears: hatred of our body, fear of being empty inside, fear of stillness, fear of being alone, fear of not being loved.
>
> (Olsen 1993, p. 48)

A generation later, dancers' mental and physical health remains an open issue. Drawing on other dance scholars who employ a Foucauldian perspec-tive, in Chapter 9 I critique contemporary dance education and professional dance practice, and make a case for using Authentic Movement to enhance and protect dancers' health and self-agency.

From movement to arts-led reflections

Visual art can have a supportive role in Authentic Movement (and in dance therapy), where it aids a transition from movement's fleeting, non-verbal mode to finding images and/or words to describe and relive those experiences.

Whilst movers enter into a profound 'silence of movement' (Sheet-Johnson 2019), movements' inherent speechlessness can find representation in visual art making. In the early days of the practice, Adler responded to what she had witnessed in her students' movements through visual art.

> I place the clay sculptures I made for each one of my students in a circle in the small studio downstairs, awaiting their arrival. Each piece is formed by my experience as a witness of their movement.
>
> (Adler 1995, p. 41)

Despite its primary conveyance in therapy and mysticism, Authentic Movement stands out amongst embodiment practices as delivering a transferable and unique method; one that combines valuable creative, embodied, spoken and collaborative elements in a cohesive form. Its key activities are moving, observing and speaking. Conceiving of Authentic Movement as an artistic, phenomenological practice, Part II of this book explores some of its aspects and qualities through making visual art. These transpositions aim to crystallise non-verbal, visual qualities of Authentic Movement for outsiders; for non-participants.

A visual artist's eye can be compared to a witness's eye: both are still, attentive, open and often empathetic towards their subject matter. Two arts essays, Chapters 4 and 6, contextualise reflections on Authentic Movement through the making and installation of art in different media and on different scales. They consider the artist's associative, contextual, emotional and haptic processes when making. Chapter 5 follows a different, more complex, critical discourse. Using the term choreomania as a starting point it thinks through collective body practice and a digital film practice in tandem. Honing in on precipitous edges of liminal states in Authentic Movement practice, it weaves descriptions of altered states, emotions and movement figurations that occur in a long circle. How can filming be made ethical, respectful and safe when, at first sight, doing so might be reminiscent of a Foucauldian surveillance? How can it not evoke notions of colonial anthropology? Describing the adaptation of ethical guidelines in a digital camera-witnessing, I consider the film *Long Circle* as an art-ethnographic document and place public audiences into the role of meta-witnesses and/or learners.

With digital photography and filming becoming ever more accessible and popular, an increasing occularcentricity of digital media can be a distraction from being present and embodied. The term camera-witnessing (Goldhahn 2007) arises from Adler's question of *Who is the Witness?* and describes a working with film that considers witness/camera and mover/filmed relationships. Questions surrounding the topic of being seen digitally are also raised in Chapter 8 in terms of the question of a digital 'authenticity' and continue in 10 and 11, when principles of camera-witnessing are applied to collaborative choreography and online sessional work that use the body in movement.

Authentic Movement's emergence as its own field

As Authentic Movement grew, a grass roots publication *A Moving Journal, Ongoing Expressions of Authentic Movement* emerged in 1996 and ceased publication in 2004. Creating its own specific forum, it became a place of exchange for a growing community and a multiplicity of practitioners' voices. Edited by Annie Geissinger, Paula Clements Sager and Joan Webb, the journal was published three times a year. Issues focused on particular aspects of Authentic Movement such as Art, Religious Practice, Sound and Therapy, publishing practitioners' poems, photos, drawings and adverts for Authentic Movement groups alongside longer articles. *A Moving Journal* celebrated its dedication to a developing practice.

Authentic Movement was also the umbrella term used by the Authentic Movement Institute in the USA offering:

> an innovative curriculum, experiential and theoretical, exploring the inter-weaving of the creative, psychological and sacred through the unique body-based process of Authentic Movement.
>
> (Haze N., Stromsted T., Adler J., Chodorow J. and
> Stewart L.H., 1996/97)

Its curriculum promised students coursework in which

> one develops kinaesthetic awareness, gaining access and giving creative expression to the inner life through an approach in which "movement" is the personality made visible.
>
> (Haze N., Stromsted T., Adler J., Chodorow J. and
> Stewart L.H., 1996/97)

In the second year of *The Moving Journal*, an open letter by Adler, Chodorow, Haze and Stromsted assured the community that Authentic Movement would escape trademarking and remain openly available (Adler, J., Chodorow, J., Haze, N., & Stromsted, T. 1997). The journal, the trainings and the announcement of non-protectionism will have all contributed to an increasing popularity of Authentic Movement. Seen in retrospect, they might have also, entirely unintentionally, contributed to the practice's increasing appropriations. Further Chodorow pointed out that Jung considered active imagination, the root concept of Authentic Movement, as

> much more than a specific meditative procedure or expressive technique. In the deepest sense, active imagination is the essential, inner-directed symbolic attitude that is at the core of psychological development.
>
> (Chodorow 1997, p. 17)

Whilst Chodorow addressed perhaps a specialised Jungian analytic and psychotherapeutic community, Patrizia Pallaro offered the growing Authentic Movement community a bundling of Adler's, Chodorow's and Starks Whitehouse's essays in one volume (Pallaro 1999), making these three proponents' thinking easily available. Hence an oscillation seemed to have taken place between establishing resources, providing a place for Authentic Movement's community to freely exchange ideas and a drive towards a more refined practice. It is typical for new methods to develop different strands, that eventually become represented by different proponents. The problem that Authentic Movement faces today, is its often incomplete absorption into different practices and therapies. However, perhaps this poses renewed opportunities for dance and other art forms? Part IV of this volume explores such departures.

The Discipline of Authentic Movement

By 2001 Adler had been teaching Authentic Movement for almost a decade in Europe, increasingly building her own, very specific practices. Her ways of working were suitable for annual, meditative, self-reflective large group retreats. These retreats were not therapy or self-help groups, but teaching retreats for developing embodied knowledge and self-reflection, where participants had to take mature responsibility for their own inner state of being. Emerging from the diadic model of the ground form, Adler developed a transpersonal discipline for groups with a new, progressive structure creating her own terminology and rituals. Adler's adaptation of respectful languaging from percept language became an equal partner to the movement experience itself. Many participants in these groups in Europe and in the USA applied what they learnt from Adler to their own therapy and teaching practices. In accordance with Adler, they called this The Discipline of Authentic Movement. Further Adler coined and defined the term in her primer *Offering from a Conscious Body, The Discipline of Authentic Movement* (Adler 2002). She structured her method in terms of the individual body, the collective body and the conscious body. Individual body describes the journey of embodiment and self-reflection that an individual participant engages in as a mover. It involves a commitment to enter the practice with a trained guide and witness and focuses on a journey from developing mover consciousness and then, as this progresses, witness consciousness. A mover works together with a teacher/witness for an extended period of time using the ground form and evolves through various stages towards being a witness herself. Further, when mover consciousness and witness consciousness have been established, collective body work develops a group practice that arises from the primary dyadic model. In group formats all participants act as movers and witnesses at different times. Personal agendas are at times rendered secondary to collective needs. Choice and surrender, individual and collective fuel the dynamic between individual and group. Movers and witnesses always act and speak as owners of their own experiences, incorporating individual responses with empathetic ones and with an awareness of the collective topos.

Developed on the back of Adler's teaching retreats, the great achievement of the Discipline of Authentic Movement, as I understand it, is its cohesiveness of a progressive method that enables meta-experiences of embodiment and language that can be used in groups. Adler gave a growing community a primer to these specific developments. She placed her work in a mystical context and the style of writing that she chose can be considered consistent with her intention to protect the discipline from easy grasp. Written in the poetic style of a teaching diary, it can remain hermetic to newcomers and researchers without any practical experience. They may find it difficult to form a coherent picture of the practice's methodology. Further, as mysticism can be felt to be beyond reproach, it can be difficult to formulate a constructive critique. How can we speak or write about Authentic Movement critically? Chapter 3 provides an open glossary, a Guide to Practice, for readers and researchers and Part III of this volume explores critical questions regarding 'authenticity'.

In the same year as Adler's primer was published, *Contact Quarterly* dedicated a special issue to Authentic Movement with contributions that referenced its early, current and potential relationships with dance, the public in visual performance and even with science, opening a widening field of enquiry (*Contact Quarterly* 2002). Concurrently, Richard House, a UK psychotherapist and thinker, proposed a deconstruction of profession-centred therapy aiming to dissolve the hierarchy between client and psychotherapist (House 2003), a discourse that he later expanded on (House 2010). In my reading of Adler, conceptual foundations for establishing non-hierarchical relationships, such as qualities of acceptance and equality, run through her writing. Based on a developmental model of a learner advancing through various stages of being seen and seeing, Adler specifies that all participants learn to be movers and witnesses. In group practices each participant discloses and shares in equal measure, the collective body (Adler 2002).

Western societies' need to rediscover collectivity and collaboration are perhaps the reason behind an appropriation of The Discipline of Authentic Movement into new and widening fields. Sox Sperry's and Lisa Tsetse's work with community long circles (Sperry & Tsetse 2003 & Tsetse 2007) described such a departure. Using elements of the Discipline of Authentic Movement, they created circles for non-violent community action outside of the 'white box' of the studio or therapy space introducing an artistic and political application. Their work seems to anticipate House's post-professional era and put it into action. Part IV of this volume takes Authentic Movement beyond therapy and mysticism, into collaborative fields in dance education, dance studies, art and ecology.

MoverWitness

In the contexts of dance therapy as well as in alternative, interdisciplinary practices, I have wrangled with the term 'authentic'. What is authentic? Is the name Authentic Movement consistent with the method? In Part III of this volume critical theories are employed to explore Authentic Movement's name and I ask if 'authentic' can be an appropriate term for the practices. Some practitioners might think of this question as contentious, even sacrilegious. My analysis and reflections have given rise to an alternative term, the phenomenologically descriptive MoverWitness.

Both essays in Part III were previously published in journals in the USA, Germany and the UK (Goldhahn 2009a, 2010a, 2015), and therefore there is some unavoidable overlap in content. They are both included here because they provide critical reflections for the community, newcomers and researchers, and may serve as a springboard for further research into Authentic Movement's philosophical concepts and ontology.

Concurrent with the publication of Pallaro's new collection of essays by 42 practitioners and proponents, *Authentic Movement: Moving the Body, Moving the Self, Being Moved* (Pallaro 2007), I completed an arts-led PhD on The Discipline of Authentic Movement titled *Shared Habitat, the MoverWitness Paradigm* (Goldhahn 2007). Pallaro's edition confirmed Authentic Movement's remit as overwhelmingly belonging to healing, psychotherapy and mystical experiences; whilst my own research focused on widening fields outside of the studio and therapy room. Coining the term MoverWitness for Authentic Movement's 'disciplined' structured practices, my research referenced primarily the arts and critical theories and posed arts-led questions. Part IV of this volume hones in on new and potential applications of Mover-Witness in dance education, training, collaboration, on-screen movement work and ecology. There are additional fields, such as phenomenology, social and natural sciences, that could also benefit from MoverWitness's practices. Focused on the joint journey of movers and witnesses in developing new skills of bodily knowledge and detailed first person verbal recall, Mover-Witness shares similarities with an emerging, embodied phenomenology.

> I look to authentic movement as a discipline where all disparity can manifest and where all that we are and are becoming can be moved. The practice itself asks me to question its relationship to this world and to explore its power as a force that can support the development of personal and global conscience.
>
> (Tsetse 2007, p. 406)

Personal and global consciences underpin a willingness to view others without judgement and to accept different viewpoints. It leads to an understanding of the individual as part of a collective. Collective body work, as described in Chapter 5, provides bodily experiences of such group belonging and intimacy. Conscious interconnectivity can lead to collaboration. Artistic collaboration is the central theme in Chapter 10 of this volume, authored equally with Soili Hämäläinen and Leena Rouhiainen, two Finnish choreographers, dancers, educators and scholars. A leaderless doing and thinking together emerges, where each viewpoint is valued. This trajectory continues in the non-dual perspective described in an ongoing interdisciplinary project in Chapter 12. Applying aspects of MoverWitness together with scientists, nature and places, this essay considers a sharing of habitats and time, exploring and challenging perceptions of the hierarchical relationship between humans and plants.

MoverWitness builds on the foundation of a democratic, non-dualistic and post-modern concept that potentially dissolves the expert/client relationship into one of equals who take turns with each other. It is exciting and useful when used in the arts, performance and science contexts. By way of this name, new applications, beyond the original therapeutic or mystical remits, open up. In contrast to existing literature on Authentic Movement I have focused less on movers' experiences and more on method and witnessing. Inevitably autobiographical material weaves through this volume. In keeping with the practice's workings, I believe that experiences are most clearly expressed when spoken by the person herself. As Mervi Juntunen poignantly states in the film *So we are here now* "My feelings are my own and no one else's" (Goldhahn 2009).

In more recent years a protectionism of teaching Adler's The Discipline of Authentic Movement has caused bewilderment amongst established teachers of the Discipline, as well as confusion to newcomers to the practices. Whilst Adler mentions the term MoverWitness, she repurposes the mandorla, an early religious icon, reinforcing sacredness as the prime goal of her practice (Adler 2015). Sacredness is also expected to form the trajectory of her forthcoming collection of essays, to be published at a similar time as this volume. Seen from my perspective today and to avoid confusion with MoverWitness, it is probably best to maintain the original label for Authentic Movement's established uses in dance therapy and in Adler's teachings of mysticism, ie. 'Authentic Movement' and 'The Discipline of Authentic Movement' respectively.

MoverWitness provides a model of becoming and for being together within a level, democratic playing field. Including both the transpersonal and the political, my work embraces non-duality but is situated within a profane, phenomenological, ecological rationale of embodied shared habitats. Coming to Authentic Movement summarises the where, when and how of Authentic Movement's workings and how my questions arose. The subsequent parts in this volume open a widening field, one in which critical theories and dance research are employed to apply the MoverWitness to diverse disciplines. My hope is for these other disciplines to benefit from an exquisite freedom to move, an acute perceptiveness of observation and meticulous, phenomenological languaging skills. In order to apply these qualities and skills, we have to let go of a name that can appear outdated and insufficiently descriptive. It is hoped that this collection of essays may inspire other creatives to employ MoverWitness as a platform for embodied, phenomenological knowing and understanding.

References

A Moving Journal. (1996–2004). Retrieved from http://www.movingjournal.org/

Adler, J. (1987). Who is the witness, a description of authentic movement. *Contact Quarterly*, Volume 12, no 1, Winter 1987, (pp.20-29).

Adler, J. (1995). *Arching backward, the mystical initiation of a contemporary woman.* Inner Traditions, Rochester, Vermont.

Adler, J. (2002). *Offering from the conscious body: the Discipline of Authentic Movement.* Inner Traditions, Rochester, Vermont.

Adler, J. (2015). The mandorla and the Discipline of Authentic Movement. *Journal of Dance & Somatic Practices*, 7: 2, (pp. 217–227).

Adler, J. (2019). Panel 1, Somatics Festival 2019, A.P.E.@ Hawley and The School For Contemporary Dance & Thought with Historic Northampton, Northampton Open Media, and the Smith College Department of Dance, 19-23 September 2019, video of conference proceedings. Online at https://vimeo.com/383359664 [last visited 2 August 2022].

Adler, J., Chodorow, J., Haze, N., Stromsted T., Stewart, L. H. (1996). Authentic Movement Movement Institute, Brochure 1996/97.

Adler, J., Chodorow, J., Haze, N., & Stromsted, T. (1997). Open letter. *A Moving Journal*, Vol. 4, No. 3, (1997), (p 9).

Bainbridge Cohen, B. (2005). *Sensing, Feeling, and Action: the experiential anatomy of Body-Mind Centering.* Wesleyan University Press, Connecticut.

Banes, S. (1993). *Democracy's Body, Judson Dance Theatre, 1962–1964.* Duke University Press, Durham and London.

Chodorow, J. (1991). *Dance therapy & depth psychology, the moving imagination.* Routledge, London.

Chodorow, J. (1997). *C.G. Jung, Jung on active imagination, key readings selected and introduced by Joan Chodorow.* Routledge, London.

Chodorow, J, (2005). Note to Eila Goldhahn, October 2005, Bern.

Contact Quarterly, a vehicle for moving ideas. Special Issue: Authentic Movement. Vol. 27, No. 2, Summer/Fall 2002.

Goldhahn, E. (2007). *Shared habitats, the MoverWitness paradigm [Doctoral dissertation, Dartington College of Arts and University of Plymouth, UK].*

Goldhahn, E. (2009a). Is authentic a meaningful name for the practice of Authentic Movement? *American Journal of Dance Therapy.* Volume 31, Issue 1, (pp. 53–64).

Goldhahn, E. (2010a). The MoverWitness exchange: interdisciplinary pedagogy and communication tool, towards an embodied and empathetic laboratory. *Conference proceedings,* Kinesthetic Empathy: Concepts and Contexts, The Watching Dance Project, *Manchester University* (22–23 April, 2010).

Goldhahn, E. (2015). Towards a new name and ontology for the Discipline of Authentic Movement. *Journal of Dance & Somatic Practices*, 7: 2 (pp. 273–285).

House, R. (2003). *Therapy beyond modernity: deconstructing and transcending profession-centred therapy*. Karnac Books, London.

House, R. (2010). *Against and Beyond Therapy: Critical essays towards a post-professional era*. PCCS Books, Ross-on-Wye.

Olsen, A. J. (1993). Being seen, being moved, authentic movement and performance. *Contact Quarterly*, Volume18, No. 1, (pp. 46–53).

Pallaro, P. (ed.) (1999). *Authentic Movement: essays by Mary Starks-Whitehouse, Janet Adler and Joan Chodorow*. Jessica Kingsley, London and Philadelphia.

Pallaro, P. (ed.) (2007). *Authentic Movement, moving the body: moving the self, being moved, a collection of essays, Vol 2*, Jessica Kingsley, London.

Payne, H. (2003). Authentic Movement, groups and psychotherapy. *Self and society – forum for contemporary psychology*, Summer 2003, volume 31, No. 2, (pp. 32–36).

Skinner, J. (2004). *The Skinner Release Technique®*, Skinner Releasing [Online]. [Accessed 15 August 2021]. Available from: http://www.skinnerreleasing.com/

Sperry, S. & Tsetse, L. (2003). Self and other, the practice of community long circle. *A Moving Journal*, Volume 10, No. 1, Spring, 2003, (pp. 3–9).

Stromsted, T. (2007a). The dancing body in psychotherapy: Reflections on Somatic psychotherapy and *Authentic Movement. Pallaro, P. (ed.) (2007) Authentic Movement, moving the body, moving the self, being moved: a collection of essays, Vol 2*. Jessica Kingsley, London, (pp.202-220).

Tetse, L. (2007). Moving the outer rim in: *Authentic Movement and nonviolence. In Pallaro, P. (ed.) (2007). Authentic Movement, moving the body, moving the self, being moved, a collection of essays, Vol 2*. Jessica Kingsley, London, (pp. 406-413).

Weir, J. (1975). The personal growth laboratory: the Laboratory Method of Changing and Learning: theory and application. *Science and Behaviour Books*. Benne, K., Bradford, L.P., Gibb, J.R., Lippitt, R.D. (eds.), Palo Alto, California.

Chapter 2

A personal narrative

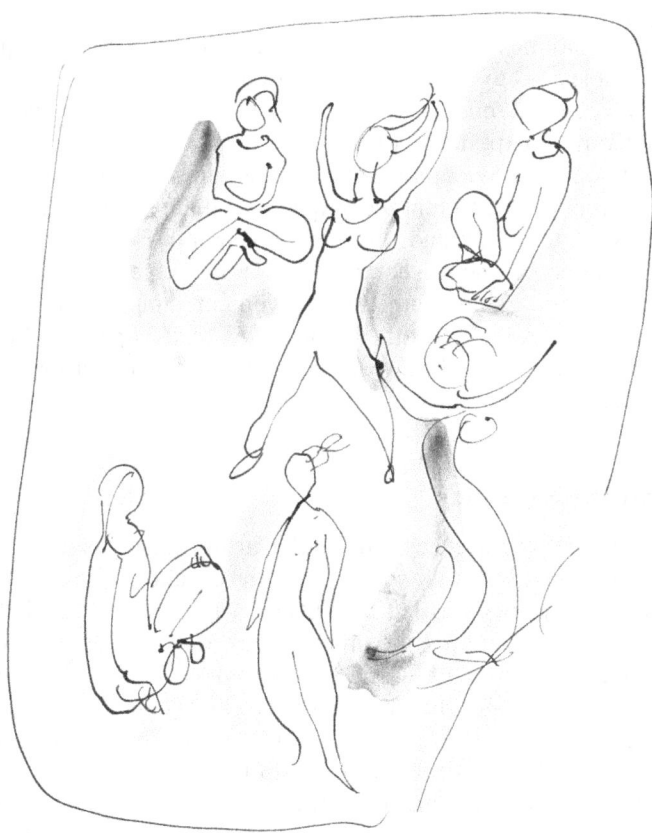

Figure 2.1 The MoverWitness: movers and witnesses, ink drawings.
Artist: Lydia Corbett, 2010.

DOI: 10.4324/9781003222309-3

Barefoot dancing

As a child I compensated a certain anxiousness with several things: I observed and connected to the natural life around me, I made things and I moved and danced in the garden at the back of our house. As childhood often foretells what is to come later in life, I created my own movement ritual in nature. I imagined the setting sun to be my witness and that this was God watching over me. A similar experience of being seen as one is, the condition and precursor to benevolent self-reflection, lies at the heart of Authentic Movement practice.

Creative dance, movement and eurythmics, according to the teachings of Jacque-Dalcroze and Carl Orff, formed part of my primary education. I loved my teacher's sessions, particularly when Frau Reuter guided us with imaginative narration into dance improvisations. At the end of each session, she would play a soft and undulating melody on her recorder to which we children wandered and meandered through the hall. As the tune grew quieter, we found our own spaces to lie down. We closed our eyes and rested while the tune found its peaceful ending. Frau Reuter's inspired rhythmical education was my first formal experience of dance.

The following narrative approximately spanning twenty years from 1980 to 2000, describes how different techniques and methods have influenced my understanding of the body and mind in movement. These methods closely touch upon contemporaneous confluences of movement, philosophy, psychology, performance and Authentic Movement and include descriptions of my studies with Adler and other proponents in Europe. On this journey, I have been inspired by and draw upon the teachings of various influential teachers as well as colleagues and students.

Voice and movement

After some painful experiences with ballet in my teens, as a young adult I became involved in Berlin's experimental dance and theatre scene. I took part in a series of workshops led by Theatergruppe Stimme und Bewegung with Vladimir Rodzianko and the architect and dancer Cornelia Hirschfeld. Rodzianko had worked with London Contemporary Dance Theatre The Place as a composer and choreographer. He also taught voice production and, in London in 1973, created Mass, a choreography in which dancers moved and sang. Hirschfeld had been a student of Mary Wigman and had developed her own teaching practice into a "playful learning of body awareness" (Bodmer 1981, p. 6), one that also encompassed movement and voice. She created specific short movement sequences around living and inert motives. Seen from today's perspective, I would describe these as "becoming-animal" (Deleuze & Guattari 2004), becoming-plant and becoming-object. In these vignettes the voice was enabled by movement and vice versa and each mirrored a specific imaginative character. Further, Rodzianko developed a method in which the production of specific consonants and vowels related to specific parts of the body (Melzian 1976). These movement techniques, like others emerging around that time, can be seen to have been defiant of ballet's ontology of silent, gravity-defying upward grace, as noted by Lepecki (2006). Stimme und Bewegung's vocabulary, whilst prescribed, was earthy, enjoyable, creative, crazy and often emotional. I experienced the joy of exploring movement and voice enhancing each other with no external stimulus of music. I felt alive and part of a multidisciplinary, creative peer community that fostered my longing to work with performance. A welcome antidote to my academic studies, I soon joined Stimme und Bewegung's performance group meeting Dartington College of Arts students at Scheersberg International Theatre Festival in 1979. I was eager to make movement and dance my professional field. Yet, despite strong traditions of dance in West Berlin and West Germany, I could not find any professional dance training, other than ballet, in my home country at that particular time. I then made the momentous decision to study abroad at Dartington, Devon, UK.

In 1978, Wigman was already 92 years old and had closed her studio in West Berlin ten years prior. Amongst the many creatives who, like Hirschfeld, had studied with Wigman was Starks Whitehouse, teacher to both Adler and Chodorow, Authentic Movement's later proponents. Like Hirschfeld, also Starks Whitehouse had integrated Wigman's work into her own personal approach to dance movement. She named this 'movement in depth' which later became 'Authentic Movement' (Starks Whitehouse, in Pallaro 1999). Wigman, Hirschfeld, Starks Whitehouse, Chodorow and Adler all considered that the sourcing of dance movement can be an entirely independent, creative act from that of listening to and being inspired by music. They believed in the moving imagination inherent in the body-mind itself. They shared this understanding with a simultaneously emerging eastern European theatre and, unbeknown to me at the time, with an American, post-modern dance, the Judson Dance Theatre, whose influences I would encounter at Dartington College of Arts, a year or so after my first encounter with Dartington students at Scheersberg.

Grotowski Theatre Laboratory

During my time in Berlin, I heard about the Theatre Laboratory in Poland, then part of the Soviet bloc. Its founder was Jerzey Grotowski, an experimental theatre director and author of a seminal collection of essays and interviews, *Towards a Poor Theatre* (Grotowski 1968). Grotowski promoted physical theatre in an intimate performance space with a small audience without any of the props that create a sense of illusion in theatre. He sought to create a 'poor theatre', championing the raw power of performers' presence to communicate directly with their 'witnesses', as he referred to the audience.

Following my application to attend a Theatre Laboratory workshop, I received an invitation to participate in the experimental performance project *Tree of People*. The acceptance letter helped me to obtain the necessary visas to travel behind the Iron Curtain, separating East from West. It also prepared me for what I was to experience, stating:

> Therefore when you arrive be a part of the stream, let it be born in you, let it flow through you. To give a chance to it one must remove the obligation of productivity and approach the element of attentiveness and straightness.
>
> (Instytut Aktors Teatr Laboratorium 1979)

I was unsure what 'removing the obligation of productivity' exactly meant but I was fascinated and eager to find out. Somewhat apprehensively, I accepted the invitation and attended "the final project by the Laboratory Theatre group belonging to active culture" (Ludzi 2012). The concept behind Tree of People was the creation of movement and dramatic action out of the synergy of all participants in the present moment. In essence, this was non-directive movement on a level playing field where participants performed spontaneously with and in front of each other. Described as *stream-work* [dzieło-rzeka], it comprised a series of improvised actions by participants working under the direction of members of the group.

It was very exciting. From my arrival onwards, for two days and nights, all participants were continually immersed in a performance mode, with simple, adjacent accommodation but without any clocks or watches, and hence without any normal circadian rhythm and orientation. Very little was spoken all weekend and there were no verbal instructions. We, a group of approximately twenty participants, seemed to have arrived from all over the world and did not get to know one another, apart through moving and watching each other silently, by eye contact, improvising, sharing some food and a few hushed comments. The studio was at times candlelit but I did not know, other than by my tiredness, whether it was day or night. I watched others and moved, sometimes spontaneously, out of myself, and sometimes in response to others. Members of the Grotowski ensemble intermingled with us as equal participants in the group. They created a non-verbal input into the collective's dynamic by merit of their clear presence, manifest in wakeful eye contact and open body language. Suspended minutes of waiting and pausing, of gauging one another's positions in space were followed by sudden rushes of activity and spontaneous dramatic situations in the studio. There was running, joining, appearances and disappearances, interactions and solo moments. People crouched on the floor, lay down or stood still and watched. There was tension and at times the lack of tension. Boredom, tiredness, confusion, lucid moments and spatial and gestural meaning-making took turns with each other.

Tree of People was my first, powerful experience of entirely non-directive movement in a studio context. Paring the performative situation down to its key players, movers and witnesses, Grotowski relied on a direct relationship between actors and audience. His interest in a direct experience of relationship had conceptual parallels to a simultaneously emerging performance practice and Authentic Movement in the USA. A safe psychological space, as understood nowadays, was not always present in those years. But I was resilient and drew some lasting memories from this brief, extraordinary experience. Unbeknown to me at the time, the intensity of focus, the relationship between movers and witnesses, and the 'removal of the obligation of productivity' were ideas that I would meet again when studying post-modern dance and Authentic Movement.

Tai Chi Chuan

In contrast to Stimme und Bewegung and Grotowski Theatre Laboratory, both deeply rooted in continental Europe's expressionist traditions, I also learned a quieter and softer movement practice originating from Far Eastern Taoist culture. In West Berlin during the late 1970s, Brigitte Bergese, mother of choreographer Micha Bergese, offered gentle movement and Tai Chi Chuan sessions fused with a study of breath and self-awareness. Her own master teacher was the Chinese Gia-fu Feng who had worked with American Alan Watts and other figureheads of the emerging East/West philosophies at Esalen Institute in California. In 1973, Jane English and Gia-fu Feng translated the Tao Te Ching (Lao Tsu 1973) into English, offering ancient Chinese wisdom to a modern West hungry for the oriental and spiritual. Gia-fu Feng visited and taught in Europe during the late 1970s and early 1980s. Eastern philosophy's wise acceptance of all things permeated his and Bergese's teachings, opening up a new and more gentle view of the body in movement for me. In this new context of movement meditation, instead of performance, my body's movement was no longer a way to express, convey and communicate with an audience, but an instrument to still my mind and my emotions, opening up a path of self-acceptance, which further helped me to ground myself and to develop a quieter, less anxious nervous system.

Like the multi-limbed, animalistic experiences of Stimme und Bewegung, Tai Chi Chuan also offered becoming-animal and becoming-nature such as in movements named *Cloud Hands*, *White Crane Spreads Wings* and *Golden Rooster on One Leg*. Here movements were performed not for others but for their own meditative sake and for an inwardly perceived feedback. Tai Chi Chuan movement offered a flow, an invisible imaginative drawing and subtle boundary making in space, which I found to be both calming and aesthetically satisfying. Gia-fu Feng's teachings determined a notion of correctness because Tai Chi Chuan is a movement form which the body has to get used to and adhere to, similar to a Yoga practice. Yet there is no stasis in Tai Chi Chuan, only momentary stillness and onward flow. Tai Chi Chuan's imaginative and multifarious movement figurations teach the body and mind to centre whilst balancing in an upright position with the energy grounding itself through the pelvis, legs and feet. The mind has to focus and see itself and the body in movement, like an inner witness in Authentic Movement.

Martha Eddy (2002) observes that around the mid-century in the West, a great appropriation of Eastern health care and well-being practices into dance and dance education took place. This is a development that continues today and is further commented on in Chapter 9 of this volume. Taoism and other Eastern practices often include authoritarian teachings about the great and unchanging laws of life, yet are widely appropriated by Western practices to support individuals' privilege and longing for self-realisation. Taoism has also influenced the development of Authentic Movement, as reflected in essay titles, statements and a subtitle such as The Tao of the Body (Starks Whitehouse 1958); 'moving and being moved' (Starks Whitehouse 1958) and like the river, return to the source (Adler 1987), that sound similar to, or even are, axioms from the Tao te Ching.

Tai Chi Chuan can give form to the formless; it makes the fearful fearless. In Authentic Movement the fearful is able to create out of the formless, expressing and enduring fear. Tai Chi Chuan instills a sense of moving and being moved within a sense of liberty given shape by its forms. This dynamic, of 'freedom within form', can also serve as a preparation for the practices of Authentic Movement.

Dartington College of Arts: Dance

Determined to follow a professional path in movement and dance, I accepted a place to study BA Hons Theatre in a Social Context at Dartington College of Arts in 1980 and moved from the city of Berlin to rural Devon in the UK. The four-year course offered a curriculum in American and British postmodern dance and performance-making and their applications in community settings. It was re-educative in such profound new ways that I could not have imagined. Following an entirely different concept than my previous dance studies, these new, softer and more subtle teachings expanded and deepened my view of the body, the mind and creativity. We studied psychology (both science-based and Jungian), anthropology, sociology, design, creative writing, acting and directing, costume and prop making, and, above all, New Dance and choreography. American choreographer and dancer Mary O'Donnell Fulkerson's almost daily two-hour-long classes in release dance formed the central core of the curriculum during the first and second years. O'Donnell Fulkerson's work is best described in her own words:

> The beginnings of this work date back about fifteen years to 1965. At that time I was a student at the University of Illinois when Joan Skinner was working through her idea of applying her personalised understandings of the Alexander Technique specifically within the context of dancing. She used a process of imagery and stillness which was important to my work when coupled with the particular anatomical images and thought processes taught by Barbara Clark, student of Mabel Ellsworth Todd. Barbara's work provided a specific anatomical pedagogy for the work with imagination that Joan had begun.
>
> (O'Donnell Fulkerson 1982, p. 5)

And further,

> When I first arrived here in England I was still using the terminology of Joan's work and I called it Release. However, I ceased to use that label, around 1975, because I felt it was not necessary to fragment the already fragmented dance world with further labels. Dancing, I believed then and I still believe, is just dancing.
>
> (O'Donnell Fulkerson 1982, p. 5)

Her studies of the body in stillness and in dance movement were taken by all theatre students, whether we aspired to be dancer/choreographer, actor/director or writer for performance, which were the three different pathways within the graduate programme. Body and mind knowledge was taught together, affirming what I had until then sensed but not consciously grasped: there is no separation and that connecting to one's body is the root of all creativity. Experiencing the body in stillness and in movement formed the basis for everyone's imagination and for all creative student work. Everything else flowed, evolved and was built around O'Donnell Fulkerson's work, akin to Jung's comment that "The symbols of the Self arise from the depth of the body" (Jung 1940, p. 173).

At Dartington, O'Donnell Fulkerson's classes started with a place of stillness lying on the smooth wooden floor of the Dance School. The resting position was the first we learned and the one we returned to again and again. We soon adopted this to help us in our own individual work. Lying on the back with the knees propped up supports the pelvis, back and head. The spine can lengthen whilst the weight of the whole body giving way aids a deep relaxation of muscles and ligaments. As one allows gravity to work on the body, there can be sensations of sinking or the floor receiving one's weight. The resting position is a turning point from activity and tension towards relaxation and non-productivity. It is a preparation for new receptivity, alertness and focus that are tuned to impulses from the body and allow the imagination to arise, similar to Jung's active imagination.

> Stillness is my starting point. I remain still for a period of time and then allow thoughts to emerge from the stillness. In emerging, thoughts are made up of both movements and ideas. There is no separation of movement and idea within this process, as both are known together in a state of being. These are thoughts without words.
>
> (O'Donnell Fulkerson 1982, p. 5)

These teachings helped me to better understand the intention of Grotowski's invocation for a "removal of the obligation of productivity" (Instytut Aktors Teatr Laboratorium 1979). Taking time to partake in meditative and dream-like states allows a consciousness of sensations of body and feelings. In time, my imaginations began to bubble up of their own accord. Encouraged by O'Donnell Fulkerson's gentle voice we rested and sank and, sometimes, even fell asleep!

Slowly and repeatedly O'Donnell Fulkerson fed us anatomical and developmental movement imagery and instruction and to my amazement, new movements arose within me without me seemingly 'doing' them, let alone having to contort my body in any way whatsoever. A typical session taught by O'Donnell Fulkerson was based on her premise that an integration takes place by way of different body parts being in continual dialogue with one another and the world (O'Donnell Fulkerson 1976). This new way of approaching dance from the imagined interiority of the body was very different to the expressionist tradition I had studied in Germany with Stimme und Bewegung. Over time, it gently softened my body and soul, uniting muscle with mind, to paraphrase Yvonne Rainer (Wood 2007). This new way of moving gave me a new privilege rooted in acceptance of my body: a bodily knowledge based in the sensory and haptic experiences of dancing. Following my body's impulses for movement was good enough. Infused by anatomical insight and meditations on physical movement and spatial principles, I felt new energy, strength and flexibility, a grace accompanied by a lessening self-consciousness. It felt like there was a matter of factness associated with dance, a reality of the body, a being rather than having a body. The question of 'authenticity' did not arise; the postmodern pragmatic wisdom of the body sufficed as its own powerful revelation.

O'Donnell Fulkerson's work was complemented by Steve Paxton's teachings in Contact Improvisation and Rosemary Butcher's in choreography.

Many more influential new dance proponents than I can mention in this book visited and taught. Paxton explained the differences that

> in the older [dance] traditions emotional projection is a primary quality. Through the technical movement, ultimately, what they are trying to do is to convey an emotional narrative. In contact and post-modern dance emotional narrative projection is seriously questioned.
>
> (Paxton 1981b)

This statement by Paxton clearly elucidated to me at the time where I had culturally come from and where I was now going.

Butcher's teaching was sensitive and highly artistic and more complex than I can fully pay tribute to here. But in this context I must mention Butcher's emphasis on teaching choreography through taking much time to look: not just observing dancers in the studio, but also witnessing everyday, pedestrian movement of individuals or group configurations in social contexts, outside in the landscape and in architecture. As well as this attention to pedestrian movement, she told me about "the spaces *between* movers, spaces and things" (Butcher 1982). My witnessing and appreciation of the beauty of configurations between movers and objects, the fall of light and shadows, this way of seeing and of art-making, stems from her teaching and performances and her aesthetic concerns.

Both Butcher and Paxton spoke to us about the different perspectives that individuals within one audience have of the same performance. This was made apparent in the different ways in which both seated their audiences, for example in the round. Paxton encouraged "to witness the action, to use your mind as a lens and witness the action, the emotions and the imagistic world as a unit" (Paxton, S. 1981b). Drawing parallels between Contact Improvisation and Grotowski's work, he pointed out that in both an audience closely witnesses intimate contact between performers (Paxton, S. 1981b).

Post-modern dance can be a a preparation for coming to Authentic Movement: stillness, listening to the body, bodily knowledge, access to the imagination and witnessing are all qualities and activities essential to Authentic Movement. These qualities deepen the ability to listen to body and mind, through the study of the body's anatomy in movement at the same time as using the imagination and preparing the mind for its imaginative journeys. Release dance is rooted in the sensory and imaginative levels of the body-mind. By processing and practicing anatomical information and simple developmental movement, easy transitions from the rational mind to the sensations of the body and its movements are created. "An imagined journey begins with the feeling of axial movement in the body" (O'Donnell Fulkerson 1976). The axial movement relates to the spine, the central core of the body, where all movement originates from and when returning to stillness ebbs. It is the beginning of movement and the return to one's core that literally centres a person in their bodily knowing.

Contact Improvisation concentrates on using one point of contact between two partners. It also utilises physical principles such as falling, rising and centrifugal force, as form- and energy-giving forces, that are engaged with playfully. Whilst standing still and observing the balancing reflexes and centring forces within the body is the starting point, Contact Improvisation is also informed by sensations of touch and kinaesthetics. Paxton describes his partner in Contact Improvisation in this way: "She doesn't direct herself – she starts moving and then lets it happen. Finding ways to cope with momentum and gravity" and, using words very similar to Starks Whitehouse, Paxton also speaks about Contact Improvisation as "moving and being moved" and that "specific movements are unpredictable" with the proviso "they occur within a knowable field – of gravity, centrifugal force, support and dependency" and "Standing became one of our disciplines, keeping the mind attentive to the body's present moment" (Paxton 1988 pp. 38-39).

At that time, Dartington College of Arts' mission built on interdisciplinarity between the arts and a grounding of creativity in and through the body. Adjacent to the dance school at Dartington was a large music studio for orchestral practice and housing the Gamelan instruments. At the time this room also hosted private training for teaching the Alexander Technique. Arts students of all disciplines (music, theatre and visual art) were welcome to participate in free lessons with students of the Alexander Technique. The anatomical learning that I received in dance was reinforced in this practice of alignment in everyday movement. Gentle touch helped to identify inner skeletal-muscular balances and alignment, alleviating some of the tensions and exertions resulting from the demands of dancing.

At Somatics Festival (2019), Nancy Stark-Smith, key proponent of Contact Improvisation and founder of *Contact Quarterly* magazine, pays tribute to the historic connections and roots between new dance, Contact Improvisation, Authentic Movement and Body Mind Centering®:

> The works were interweaving through the people, who were finding them and finding each other, and moving to different places, so I feel that the magazine [Contact Quarterly], almost like a person, had a role in that.
>
> (Starks-Smith, 2019, min 43)

Influenced by a small international network, Dartington was the first place in Europe to receive the teachings of the post-modern dance practices by their foremost proponents.

Dance therapy and Authentic Movement

After graduation, I taught body awareness, creative dance and Tai Chi in local communities, hospitals and day centres around South Devon. Seeking to deepen my practice I also connected with the Association of Dance Movement Therapy UK and undertook a training in client-centred, Rogerian counselling, an approach to verbal therapy which has much in common with the practice of mirroring in dance therapy. Mirroring in dance therapy can strengthen a client's identity by their movements being offered back to them. Essentially the therapist or counsellor only reflects back to the client what they have heard the client say or seen her move and no interpretation or analysis is offered.

Dance therapy as a profession was emerging in the UK as dance movement therapy with Lynn Crane, Catalina Garvie and Helen Payne (as chair) initially spearheading the new professional association. I attended professional development workshops in London with American dance therapy teachers Marcia Leventhal, Joanna Gerwetz Harris and others. Whilst I gained valuable insights and knowledge of different approaches to creative and expressive dance therapy in groups, I longed to find a method in dance therapy that would more fully echo and expand what I already knew. Through my training at Dartington, I had already gathered a deep knowledge of body, mind and creativity in movement and interdisciplinary arts that deserved to be built on directly. Then three synchronistic events shaped my further journey.

I read Adler's seminal article "Who is the Witness, A Description of Authentic Movement" (Adler 1987). Her notion of the mover and witness being together on a conjoined journey resonated deeply with my search and knowing. At various stages in my life and movement training, I had felt witnessed and Adler's description of the mover's and witness's journeys in Authentic Movement echoed my experiences of performative and therapeutic situations. At the same time, as ringing deeply true, Adler's descriptions opened new questions for me: How could a witness ever be without judgement? How was the beauty of what was seen created? Was this practice an art form or was it dance therapy? How could I apply this in my sessions? And who was Adler and what had enabled her to have such insights and clarity?

Then, only a couple of weeks after reading Adler, a stranger rung me out of the blue and introduced herself as Wendy Elliott, an American dance therapist. She had seen my flyer advertising movement classes locally and wanted to connect with me. She was on a sabbatical year in a neighbouring village. She practiced something called Authentic Movement (!) and did I want to meet her? Yes, I did! For the following six months or so, Elliot and I met regularly. She had been part of Adler's second cohort of The Mary Starks Whitehouse Institute in 1982 and in addition, had received individual tuition and supervision from Adler. Elliott introduced me to the ground form of Authentic Movement: the dyadic exchange between a mover and a witness, and my Authentic Movement training began here. Working one-to-one with Elliott was a privilege, as was the freedom to go beyond any notion of intentionality of movement. Whilst reminiscent of a meditation or a Tai Chi practice, but without a formal movement language, Elliott as my witness would give me her undivided focus and attention paired with a very special loving kindness, la benevolencia. Whilst I was well familiar with stillness, anatomy, Newton's laws of motion and my own imagination, the mantra of letting go into being moved now encompassed a wider, more open and warmer field of exploration and surprise. Being trained in New Dance had focused on the proprioceptive senses, on the joy and sensation of my movements in space. Authentic Movement gave me yet a wider field of feeling qualities and gestures, to simply reveal myself to myself and my witness, without seeking out the thrill of my dancing.

Learning to be a witness in Authentic Movement was not easy. Observing Elliott's movement, I was confronted with a new awareness of myself, namely that of my judgement of another's movement. As I became more conscious of this, I also realised how this attitude had, in part, been formed by my previous dance training. Even the soft and libertarian approaches of contemporary post-modern dance, Release and Contact improvisation had left inscriptions, not just on my body's preferential movements, but also on my perceptions of others' dance movement. I had been taught to make economical use of energy and effort and to control my weight when running, falling, rising up from and sinking into the floor or when spinning and rolling, in keeping with O'Donnell Fulkerson's ideas. Whilst O'Donnell Fulkerson's teaching had enabled me to find much liberation and access to my movement and creativity, moving 'properly' now stood in the way of my non-judgmental looking at others. With the knowledge of anatomical imagery and effortless flow, my training had imbued me with a distinct aesthetic that I habitually applied to see movement. I found 'awkward' movement, that didn't make the best ergonomic use of the body, more difficult to accept and to witness. However, confronting and accepting my imperfect witnessing brought its own useful insight. Movement flow and gravity-using and gravity-defying grace, impressed upon me as qualities of dance movement in Release Dance, are not necessarily present in Authentic Movement. Authentic Movement instead is sourced from a reality of the body and mind in movement that includes starkness, stagnation and awkwardness as well as lighter flowing forms of movement. When learning the witnessing part of Authentic Movement, I needed to address my preconceptions that had guided my own movement and my perceptions of others' movement. It also meant to accept my own boredom at times.

Studying Authentic Movement with Elliott reminded me of some of the earthy and idiosyncratic animal-becomings such as those I had performed in Stimme und Bewegung. Harking back to this earlier, expressionist movement training helped me to open up wider and deeper movement ranges within myself. I began to source and to witness movements that had been somewhat blindsided from my dance vocabulary as a post-modern dancer.

My inner witness began to expand and to relax into a more permissive and non-judgemental state. By the time Elliot left the UK, I had integrated the ground form of Authentic Movement and began to use it in my own teaching. I melded exercises and improvisations from Tai Chi, Release Dance and Contact Improvisation as preparations for working with Authentic Movement.

On a summer's day, another unexpected event took place. I found a lost book on a grass verge near the sea, titled *Human Nature* (Winnicott 1988). I had heard about Winnicott but had not read his original writings before. On reading, I found its contents closely corresponded to the quiet and developmental approaches to movement and the imagination that I knew and that I intuited for the kind of dance therapy I sought to practice. Winnicott had closely worked with infants and mothers, and written with great sensitivity and insight about the main issues in psychoanalysis. One of the most fascinating aspects I found to be his work on creativity in the first acts of the infant after birth and the developing individuality of the infant in the intimate relationship with a caregiver. His writing touched upon my own inner wound, an early separation trauma, and gave me understanding and comfort in my own psychotherapeutic process.

Authentic Movement with Adler, Italy

Adler's first international group retreat in the Discipline of Authentic Movement was organised by Helen Payne and Kedzie Penfield, taking place in 1992 in the UK. The following year, prompted by Elliot, I received a personal invitation to attend Adler's next European retreat in the Discipline of Authentic Movement in Italy, organised by Rosa-Maria Govoni. This group consisted of about twenty women participants from many different cultural backgrounds and many different mother tongues and accents. Everybody had a background in psychotherapy, dance therapy or dance and almost everybody was new to me. Unusually the retreat house had a tiled studio, originally two rooms now opened up into one. There were windows out to a Tuscan landscape with olive trees and a Mediterranean blue sky. We mostly worked as a whole group of movers, being observed and witnessed by Adler and Tina Stromsted, introduced as her assistant. Both were seated near the opening between the two spaces so that they could witness as much as possible. I had several challenges: to move within a crowded space, to negotiate a hard floor and to be part of a large new group, where each participant had a different movement language. I adapted my habitual movement expression to be less expansive, more careful when going down to the floor and when encountering other movers. I also learnt to actively remember my movement and I experienced longing to be seen by Adler's kind eyes. Understanding the different accents and translations from other languages into English was both a challenge and, at times, gave room for hilarity and relief from the often serious work. There were silent times akin to a meditation retreat and, like a meditation teacher, Adler would give individual witnessing outside of the studio sessions. These encounters felt very precious but they also carried tension of expectation and uncertainty. At times I felt insecure in this arrangement, not knowing when Adler might come up to me to offer me her individual attention. I entered into a powerful projection on Adler and her practice, where I experienced much longing to be seen and spoken to by her. I felt moved by Adler's countenance and composure, her witnessing and way of speaking and the feeling of her warm and wise attention resting upon me. Stromsted was in a supportive role to Adler, giving valuable contact and verbal witnessing too, but I did not experience the same projection upon her. In the group, I met Payne and Marcia Plevin and many other dance therapy colleagues and formed the beginning of lasting peer relationships. After five days, at the end of the retreat and when taking leave, I was awash with tears, feeling love and connection towards Adler. I was not the only enchanted one. At the time, I did not understand the reason behind our powerful feelings towards Adler. There was something very special and wise about her, a charismatic mystique; that she saw me how I was. When leave-taking, I shared my feelings with her. She responded in her characteristically ardent and sincere way.

The following year, in 1994, we met again with Adler and Stromsted in Italy, now in another retreat centre, La Capannace near Pisa, and this was to become our group's home for five years. The very large studio was housed in a dedicated building with a smooth wooden floor and tall windows. We would use just one-half of it as it was so huge. Over the following years, this place became the venue of many Authentic Movement retreats, not just Adler's, but also Stromsted's, who built up her own groups, and peer groups such as La Luna, organised by Celine Gimbrere. During those precious years with Adler, the profound, therapeutic potential of Authentic Movement increasingly worked upon my body and soul, whilst Adler's concepts and group practices became clear and familiar to me. Pertinent experiences of myself as a participant of this particular group formed my understanding of its therapeutic powers, its creative potential and its dangers. During these years (1993 to 1999) Adler's teaching evolved year by year. Our group's work together featured dyadic work, long circle, breathing circle and long transition times filled with thinking and reflective writing. Ritualistic elements to safeguard the work, such as walking the perimeters of the circle, conscious eye contact and 'sprouting', were developed to affirm wakeful presence and consciousness. Our speaking circles became increasingly dedicated to Adler's interpretation of percept language with elements of languaging, affirmation, echoing and silences. Silent transition times became more precious as I walked, wrote, drew and gathered natural objects that became metaphors. There were also discussion times, where we could bring questions and listen to Adler's evolving concepts interwoven with personal anecdotes in her unmistakable humorous and touching way. Once I started to study with Adler, my own teaching began to embrace percept language and I used Authentic Movement increasingly in the context of one-to-one dance therapy. Working with others and passing the work on became deeply rewarding.

In 1995, Adler's book *Arching Backwards, the Mystical Initiation of a Contemporary Woman* was published and revealed the depth and pain of Adler's experiences. At the time I found it difficult to read the content of this book and was only able to digest some passages at a time. I had, as yet, no concept of how anyone could survive such painful imagery in what were Adler's long and dark nights of the soul. I could only guess that, perhaps, Adler's survival of such experiences had given her the gifts of seeing others in the present time with intensity and love beyond the ordinarily human.

Jungian psychology

It was during the 1990s that I became involved in the Jungian study circle at Luscombe in Devon and undertook personal analysis with Julian David. Deepening my understanding of myself, I worked towards UK registration as a dance movement psychotherapist. I had been previously introduced to Jungian psychology at Dartington College of Arts where David had lectured on the subject. I had also undertaken some counselling with his wife Yasmin David. Primarily a talented poet and landscape painter, David had encouraged a reflective, creative and private approach to life, one that her husband Julian shared.

The study circle focused on fairytales and myths in relation to Jung's work. Sited within old country houses against the backdrop of the rural Devon landscape, this context enabled a quiet and deep absorption of Jungian thought, a dipping into the unconscious itself and an increasing sensibility for my own unique journey. Inadvertently, the setting also invited some (less fruitful) projections of person-centred wisdom and grandeur. Initially, I found it a challenge to bring my own bodily and creative knowledge into this study circle which was based on text, mythical narrative and telling of dreams. Through the study circle I met Anthony Stevens. A prolific author combining Jungian thought with ethological research as a psychiatrist, he inspired me to delve deeper into the relevance and meanings of archetypes, myths and the effect of environment and genetics on early attachment. After dinner readings and discussions of Stevens's work on *Private Myths: Dreams and Dreaming* (Stevens 1995) built a web of intellectual reflection and community with these Jungians. It also connected subjective knowledges, such as Jungian thought and embodiment, to ethology, on which attachment theorists, such as Winnicott and John Bolwby (Holmes 1993) had drawn. Chodorow's understanding of developmental movement from a Jungian and dance therapy perspective (Chodorow 1991) became the other theoretical context for my practice. In 1997, I received the senior registration of the UK Association for Dance Movement Psychotherapy authorising me to supervise and to train. All during this time I attended Adler's retreats in Italy at La Capanacce together with a steady nucleus of about twelve women returning year after year, as we committed to the practice. In 2000 I contributed a lecture titled "Jungian Psychology and Authentic Movement" at the Luscombe study circle by an ancient fireplace.

Authentic Movement with Adler, Greece

The last two years of Adler's teaching in Europe took place in Greece. During the 2001 retreat on Andros, Adler spoke much about the book she was writing on the Discipline of Authentic Movement and a new study aspect was encouraged in our work. We split into subgroups during the afternoons and discussed specific questions we had about her emerging discipline. These were shared each day in the plenary of the group.

> Seeking out the clarity and fierceness of its light, Adler chose the sparseness and simplicity of a Greek island to continue teaching our group the Discipline of Authentic Movement. Arriving on the Greek island of Andros in scorching sunlight and heat, so intense that being outside was unbearable during most of the hours of the day. Our studio at the very top of the building, up several flights of steps, was hot, windy and very, very light. A bare wooden square with windowed doors to all directions of the sky, where we could step out onto the roof above the constantly moving palm fronds, and where thin white cotton veils gave the illusion of the fierce sunlight being tempered on its entry to the room. Adler had changed her methods from working in a large group of twenty participants in Italy in the collective body format to working instead in two small groups of six participants each, often with a single mover being observed by all the others, I felt quite exposed to five or six pairs of eyes.
>
> (Goldhahn 2001)

In a letter, Adler had asked existing students to make a conscious choice to continue studying the 'Discipline' with her in Greece, as opposed to Italy, concurrent with her own increasing focus that demanded an intensification of the surrounding environment. Not unlike a painter, Adler sought out the best light conditions, literally emphasising the importance of clear and well-lit visuality in the practice of witnessing. Reminiscent of metaphysical meanings of light, originating from Platonic thought, Adler touched on a line of thinking which runs through Christian and Judaic mysticism, the age of enlightenment and Copernican occularcentricity. The association of light with good and darkness with evil continues to be powerfully alive today (Levin 1993; Derrida 1993).

In the Greek studio, Adler introduced a new practice format: small groups of five or six participants worked together witnessing just one person moving on their own. This was a new challenge. As a mover and as a witness, I felt more keenly exposed to what I was doing and saying. It was challenging work and I felt put on the spot as I had not felt before in my work with Adler. In the languaging part of these sessions, Adler guided us on how to dedicate our words to precisely describing the movement we witnessed. She encouraged us to select and focus on describing a small moment in time in order to reach precision. Comparing the inner process of finding the words that would match our perceptions to the peeling away of layers of an onion, we searched for ever deeper layers of experiences, reaching deeper and deeper into the insights of our own embodiment. In effect we would reflect in words upon the embodiment of the mover to become more conscious in ourselves. In moments of insight, words were found that synchronistically matched and resonated with the thoughts and feelings of the mover and those of other witnesses. Becoming conscious of oneself is the aim of Authentic Movement. Finding unity in what is expressed can create true intimacy with others, or even give rise to a unifying experience, akin to an experience of the sublime. In September 2001, the terror attacks on the World Trade Centre in New York shocked the world and I believe as a result Adler decided to no longer fly to Europe.

The following year Adler's primer *Offering from a Conscious Body, The Discipline of Authentic Movement* was published. It is a beautiful, poetic book in which she describes the workings of the practice as I had come to know it during the aforementioned retreats. It also inspired me to embark on my own research. With the written evidence of the method, practices and concept for The Discipline of Authentic Movement at hand, I found it easier to ask my own questions and to experiment with visualisations and writing. Adler had provided a springboard for me to develop my own viewpoint. Over the following years, whilst I was sad that Adler would no longer travel to Europe and without sufficient resources or will of my own to travel the long distance to Vancouver, Canada, (where she was now offering retreats), the realisation dawned on me, that I now had to stand on my own two feet. As a result, my projection on Adler lessened and this freed me to develop my own research and viewpoint on Authentic Movement.

Conclusions

Looking back, my encounter with the Theatre Laboratory introduced me to the concept of the freedom from 'the obligation of productivity'. Tai Chi was an introduction to meditation and a new aesthetic sourced in the easily flowing forms of becoming nature and animal, of 'moving and being moved', a much-repeated mantra in Authentic Movement. My four years at Dartington with O'Donnell Fulkerson was my true apprenticeship, creating lasting bodily knowledge and a place within me to return to again and again. I cannot praise her work enough. It was without comparison, rich with experiences of embodied learning without which I would not have been able to enter the practices of Authentic Movement so confidently. These were taught to me so excellently and sensitively by Elliott, Adler and Stromsted. In their ardour, personal teaching and presence they enabled me to undergo some transformative, deeply moving and profound processes. Developing empathy and communication skills through the learning of percept language built the foundation for a shared habitat of my working with others, with film and with other arts methods (Goldhahn 2007). Without these teachers and Adler's primer of the Discipline of Authentic Movement, my research could not be what it is. My gratitude.

Coming to Authentic Movement is different for everybody. A training in dance in not required, but post-modern dance can be a helpful preparation, as are meditation,Tai Chi Chuan and somatic practices. In my case, the grounding in expressionist physical theatre and post-modern dance made me look at Authentic Movement as a deeply moving art form that closely connects to Self and others. My direct experiences of some of the 20th century's key influencers in this field reveal similarities between contemporaneous disciplines, all emerging at a similar, fertile time.

References

Adler, J. (1987). Who is the witness, a description of Authentic Movement. *Contact Quarterly,* Vol. 12, No 1, (pp 20-29).

Adler, J. (1995). *Arching backward, the mystical initiation of a contemporary woman.* Inner Traditions, Rochester, Vermont.

Adler, J. (2002). *Offering from the conscious body: the Discipline of Authentic Movement.* Inner Traditions, Rochester, Vermont.

Alexander, F. M. (1931). *The use of the self.* Methuen & Co. Ltd, London.

Bodmer, F. (1981). *Stimme und Bewegung*, Diplomarbeit, unpublished. *Stimme und Bewegung.* Unpublished thesis.

Butcher, R. (1982). Rosemary Butcher in interview with Eila Goldhahn at Dartington College of Arts, UK. Unpublished course work.

Chodorow, J. (1991). *Dance therapy & depth psychology, the moving imagination.* Routledge, London.

Chodorow, J. (1997). *C.G. Jung, Jung on active imagination, key readings selected and introduced by Joan Chodorow.* Routledge, London.

Deleuze, G. & Guattari, F. (2004). Becoming-animal. Atterton, P. & Calarco, M. (eds.) *Animal philosophy.* Continuum, London, (pp. 85–100).

Derrida, J. (1993). *Memoirs of the blind, the self portraits and other ruins*. University of Chicago Press, London.

Eddy, M. H. (2002). Dance and somatic inquiry in studio and community dance programs. *Journal of Dance Education*, Volume 2, No. 4, (pp. 119–127).

Elliott, W. (2021). Email to Eila Goldhahn, 7 March 2021.

Goldhahn, E. (2001). Study diary for The Discipline of Authentic Movement with Janet Adler, Greece.

Goldhahn, E. (2007). *Shared habitats, the MoverWitness paradigm* [Doctoral dissertation, Dartington College of Arts and University of Plymouth, UK].

Goldhahn, E. (2011) *Long circle* (Film).

Grotowski, J. (1968). *Towards a poor theatre*. Odin Teatres Forlag, Denmark.

Holmes, J. (1993). *John Bowlby & attachment theory*. Routledge, London.

Instytut Aktors Teatr Laboratorium (1979). Invitation letter for *Tree of People* to E. Goldhahn, 4 July 1979.

Jung, C. G. (1940). *The psychology of the child archetype. The Collected Works of C. G. Jung* (Vol. 9, Part 1, pp. 151–181) (1969). Princeton University Press, Princeton, NJ.

Jung, C.G. (1997) *Jung on active imagination, key readings selected and introduced by Joan Chodorow*. Chodorow, J. (ed.), Routledge, London.

Kolankiewicz, L. (2012). available online https://grotowski.net/en/encyclopedia/grotowski-jerzy [last visited 18 February 2021].

Lao Tsu (1973). *Tao te ching*. Wildwood House, UK.

Levin, D. M. (1993). *Modernity and the hegemony of vision*. University of California Press, London.

Lepecki, A. (2006). *Exhausting dance, performance and the politics of movement*. Routledge, New York.

Ludzi, D. (2012). *Tree of People*. [online] Available at: https://grotowski.net/en/encyclopedia/tree-people-drzewo-ludzi [last accessed 18 February 2021].

Melzian, J. (1976). Synthesizer im Kehlkopf, *tip-Berlin*, 5/79, Berlin.

O'Donnell Fulkerson, M. (1976). *The language of the axis*. Dartington Theatre Papers, Dartington College of Arts, UK.

O'Donnell Fulkerson, M. (1982). *The move to stillness*. Dartington Theatre Papers, Dartington College of Arts, UK.

Pallaro, P. (ed.) (1999). *Authentic Movement: essays by Mary Starks-Whitehouse, Janet Adler and Joan Chodorow*. Jessica Kingsley, London & Philadelphia.

Paxton, S. (1981a). *Contact improvisation*. Steve Paxton in interview with Folkert Bents. June 1981. Dartington Theatre Papers, Dartington College of Arts, UK.

Paxton, S. (1981b). Study diary by Eila Goldhahn at Dartington College of Arts, UK. Unpublished coursework.

Paxton, S. (1988). Fall after Newton. *Contact Quarterly*, Volume 13, No. 3, (pp. 38–39).

Rodzianko, V. (1979). TSUB, Theatergruppe Stimme und Bewegung. Programm note, Tanzfabrik, Berlin.

Skinner, J. (2004). *The Skinner Release Technique®, Skinner Releasing* [Online]. [Accessed 15 August 2021]. Available from: http://www.skinnerreleasing.com/

Stark-Smith, N. (2019). Panel 1, Somatics Festival 2019, A.P.E.@ Hawley and The School For Contemporary Dance & Thought with Historic Northampton, Northampton Open Media, and the Smith College Department of Dance, 19-23 September 2019, video of conference proceedings. Online at https://vimeo.com/383359664 [last visited 2 August 2022].

Starks Whitehouse, M. (1958). *The tao of the body*. In Pallaro, P. (ed.) (1999). *Authentic Movement: essays by Mary Starks-Whitehouse, Janet Adler and Joan Chodorow*. Jessica Kingsley, London and Philadelphia.

Stevens, A. (1995). *Private myths: dreams and dreaming*, Penguin, London.

Todd, M. E. (1959). *The thinking body: a study of the balancing forces of dynamic man*. Dance Horizons, New York.

Winnicott, D. W. (1988). *Human nature*, The Winnicott Trust, London.

Wood, C. (2007). *Yvonne Rainer: The mind is a muscle*. Afterall Books, University of the Arts London, London.

Chapter 3

Authentic Movement: a guide to practice

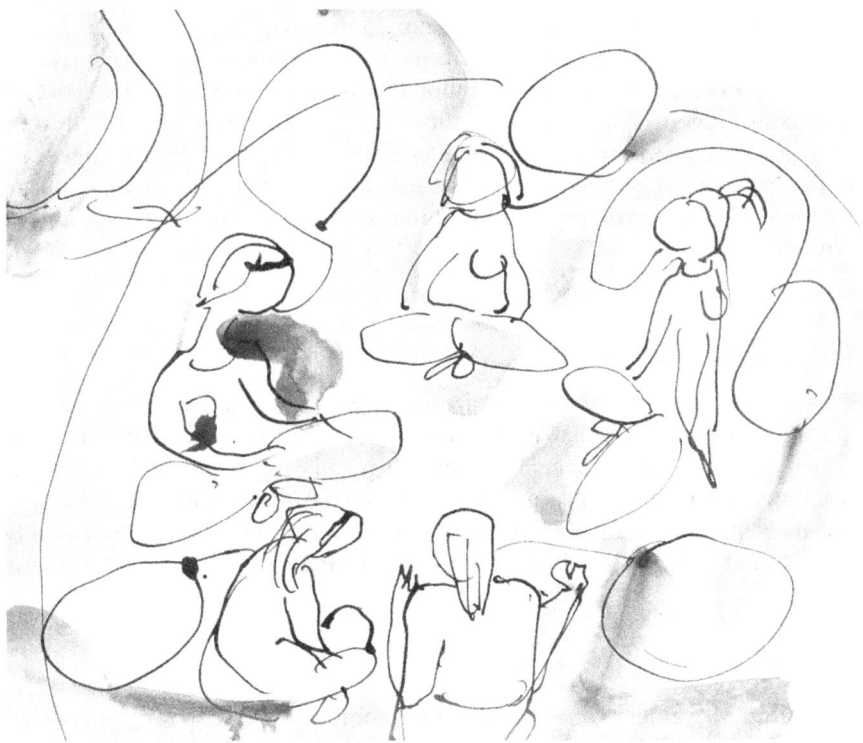

Figure 3.1 The Mover/Witness: speaking circle, ink drawings.
Artist: Lydia Corbett, 2010.

DOI: 10.4324/9781003222309-4

Introduction

This guide provides a map to the terms and practices that I and other professional practitioners use in Authentic Movement and that are referred to in other chapters of this book. Based on terminology and practices originally described in *The Discipline of Authentic Movement* (Adler 2002), this guide is aimed at researchers, students and practitioners. Placing particular emphasis on Authentic Movement's methodological framework and languaging, it is written in a pragmatic style. However, it is not a manual or a 'how to' guide; it provides definitions and explanations of practice elements and can be used by those who already practice Authentic Movement, providing additional information and reminders.

As in Chapter 1 and 9 of this volume, I emphasise the use of percept language. The craft of percept language is less known than the movement aspect of Authentic Movement, yet its skillful application has substantial benefits, including enjoyment and safety. Whilst the practice is more commonly known for the opportunity to experience embodiment and to be seen, percept language must not be missed out in any analysis and understanding of Authentic Movement. It is the other side of the coin. The guide is primarily designed around teaching and peer practices, it is not a manual for psychotherapy or self-help. Further it does not purport to be complete. An expanding guide to practice is also available on www.sharedhabitat.net

Authentic Movement

This umbrella term is used by many practitioners/teachers. It is useful for students to establish what background and tradition a teacher follows and which, if any, of the concepts described in this guide are included in their teaching. There are many groups who use the term Authentic Movement for their practice and they typically agree on a set of rules and practice formats that they will collectively abide by (Pallaro 2007).

Safe space

Authentic Movement is normally a studio practice where participants meet in each other's personal presence. The meeting space is free of intrusion or disturbance, furniture or clutter; it is private and clean. Participants leave their shoes outside of the space and bring a cushion to sit on the floor. Work takes place on the floor. If a chair is needed for comfort, then all participants should use chairs to retain spatial and visual equality.

The teacher of the practice infuses the studio space with a calm and peaceful atmosphere. She embodies the knowledge required for this practice to be safe. Prior to any sessions, she will establish by interview and/or by questionaire that participants are well, and will try to anticipate that a practice of Authentic Movement would not evoke psychological trauma. All participants need to encounter the practice safely. They need to be able to plunge their own inner depths in the presence of a teacher who has done so before them. They also need to find out whether the practice is conducive to their psychological attitude. For some, the practice is not suited or they may be not ready or interested to pursue Authentic Movement after an initial interview and session. There is no right or wrong, better or worse about a readiness to practice Authentic Movement, it simply does not suit everyone.

The psychological space in Authentic Movement is also made safe by a set of clear ethical guidelines that include:

- the movement and the dialogue between mover and witness is confidential
- the only exception to this rule is equally confidential professional supervision
- participants must not hurt themselves or others
- no physical contact between participants unless consented by both parties
- no sexual contact between participants
- mutual respect; including as to gender, race and faith
- the mover is always the expert of their own experiences
- the witness, if invited, may reflect back what the mover has spoken of.

A safe space is where individuals are respected for who they are and how they choose to be, and where they are seen and heard in an accepting, welcoming atmosphere.

The mover

The mover is one of the key players in this practice. Moving with her eyes closed in the safe space that the witness has prepared, she is granted liberty to explore the full range of her movement expressions from stillness, gentle to vigorous and all the many gestures and dynamics that may lie in between. There is no other task or frame for her than the empty space and the given time in which she can follow her impulses, to move as much or as little as she wants. From initial explorations to letting go into involuntary so-called 'authentic' movement impulses, the space is hers to fill or to leave sparse in whatever dynamic is right for her in the present moment.

Mover consciousness

Over time a participant develops consciousness of herself in movement. In Authentic Movement this is facilitated not by external direction or stimuli but by applying a focused awareness. This is used to learn to be still and to follow movement impulses with her eyes shut. To begin with this can be disorientating, but in time her bodily confidence increases, grounding her within her own physical presence and providing awareness of her own movements in space. With practice her body and mind feed back information about her body's haptic sense and her spatial orientation. Familiarity with her 'blind' motility then provides a kinaesthetic basis so she can explore her feelings, images, impulses and intuitions. These different levels of knowing all interlink with her conscious experience of her body. This coming together of body and mind adds to the often surprising insights gained through Authentic Movement. Mover consciousness is knowledge garnered through the body in motion. This will also help a mover to understand others' movement. Mover consciousness enables her to explore touch, moving together and proximity within a safe space.

The witness

The witness is the other key player in this practice. She prepares an empty and safe space, physically and psychologically. Sitting still with her eyes open she has the privilege to observe the mover. She has a double focus: her task is to be alert to both the mover and to her own self. She remains alert and gently focused on the mover. She keeps time, provides eye contact and an open-hearted presence for the mover. She is warm and welcoming. She is interested and wants to see the mover in their otherness and individuality. Her seeing and her reflections of the mover are non-judgmental and she is able to maintain silence when required.

Witness consciousness

The witness, when acting as a trainer and teacher to others, has a good understanding of the body in movement, such as alignment, muscle tone, range of movement and what is physically safe to do and what is not. She has an understanding of psychology and understands qualities of consciousness and of unconsciousness, developmental and relational psychology and psychotherapeutic process. However, when used as a peer practice not all these skills will always be present. Here the main quality of witness consciousness is the capacity to see herself and others with empathy and compassion. The witness is able to clearly distinguish between her own feelings for herself and those for others, and she has an acute kinaesthetic and intuitive sense of a safe physical and psychological atmosphere. A witness's consciousness is never perfect but she is capable of observing and recalling what the mover does without judging this. She has mastered the use of percept language and she knows when to respectfully keep silence in order to respect the mover's integrity. The witness may see and experience the mover's material without having to speak about this for her own sake. She is able to contain. She welcomes the mover in whatever way the mover needs to be.

Inner witness

The inner witness of a person is essentially an internalised view of herself formed by experience. This can range from benevolent to undermining and is initially formed by her experience of her caregivers. It is Authentic Movement's premise that the inner witness is malleable and can change. The method employed by Authentic Movement is providing a benevolent outer witness who is non-judgmental and welcoming to the mover in all her embodied expressions. The dialogue with the outer witness then provides a further blue print for an all-accepting, perceptive dialogue with one's inner witness. As a mover or witness becomes more aware of the qualities of her inner witness, an outer 'good enough' witness can be internalised. This practice is thought to overwrite past conditioning and, in time, create more inner peace and resolution.

Eye contact

Eye contact between mover and witness establishes a conscious awareness of the relationship between the two players. For the mover it also communicates her witness's commitment to be present when she subsequently closes her eyes and lets go into her inner world. It is both an expression of trust and a way to seal the contract to practice together. Authentic Movement practice can trigger an awareness of strong physical sensations, memories, feelings and images. If at any point the mover feels overwhelmed or she wants to finish her movement, she opens her eyes and re-establishes eye contact with her witness. Vice versa the witness may call the mover to end her movement phase and establish new eye contact. This could happen when there are external or internal reasons that make the witness feel unsafe. There are also instances when eye contact with the witness can be difficult, for example when feelings of shame have occurred in the mover's expressions. The mover may feel exposed and vulnerable. These can be sensitive moments for mover and witness alike. However, when contact is re-established, eye contact can be particularly poignant.

Silence

Silence is the foremost premise of the mover. Listening inward in silence her movement emerges. Her movement unfolds and is seen in silence, honouring 'the silence of movement' (Sheet-Johnson 2019).

Brief silences are held before and after movement time. They help participants to attune to each other and the practice, creating a preparation between different levels of experience and consciousness. Silence can also be used to create and to practice containment. When a new witness initially feels overwhelmed or excited by what she sees and feels, she might be compelled to tell the mover all her experiences. This can be disquieting and invasive for the mover and, in the practice of Authentic Movement, the novice witness will be encouraged to practice silence. This strengthens the mover's trust in her witness's capacity to contain the mover's and her own material safely and mindfully. As the witness learns inner witnessing through silence, the mover learns to trust and can concentrate on remembering and understanding her own material. Respect, trust and intimacy can arise between a mover and a witness when a discipline of silence and of applying percept language is kept. Mindful silence and carefully weighed words enable the benefits of Authentic Movement to emerge.

Stillness

Both mover and witness begin from a place of stillness, but whilst the mover is free to move, the witness maintains her stillness. Her place is rooted, she does not leave it and she receives the mover's material from a place of stillness within herself. The practice is meditative and provides for the expression of embodied speeds, those that help perception and focus. Stillness can relieve and disrupt overloaded minds filled by speedily moving images on screens, fast vehicular travel and a flood of differing experiences too overwhelming to be sensibly digested (Lotringer & Virilio 2005). A sense of time pervades Authentic Movement practices that, like a deep intake of breath, allow spaciousness and creativity to emerge.

Closed eyes

There is no specific term for the inner states induced by closing one's eyes whilst purposefully maintaining wakeful consciousness. It is used in prayer and meditation techniques. Phosphene is the medical term that describes the visual phenomena when no direct light reaches the visual nerve inside of the eye. Patterns and hallucinations can occur, and these have been explored in some mystical traditions and practices, such as in Tibetan Buddhism's so-called dark retreats. Moving with closed eyes undoubtedly contributes to a heightened awareness of sensations, colours, shapes and imaginations.

In Authentic Movement, as in a meditation of mindfulness, the mover closes her eyes to focus inwardly on her moving body and on any haptic, emotional, imaginative and energetic experiences that emerge. Moving with closed eyes is particularly powerful because the kinaesthetic sense is heightened. In addition, a sense of spatial disorientation can feed active imagining. It has the potential to evoke hallucinations and this is the reason why it can be unsuitable for some people, as a latent psychosis could be triggered unintentionally. Hence working in this manner always calls for due care. The recommended time period to blindly move is set in accordance with the experience of the mover, starting with a very brief period of 1–2 minutes, potentially increasing to 15–20 minutes. A gentle 'open your eyes' appeal is spoken by a witness who senses that a mover is adrift in and out of waking consciousness. This must be followed by the mover to re-establish a shared and consciously experienced reality. Further, the mover must open her eyes if she is about to move very fast, large or sudden so that her own and others' physical safety is protected. Conscious awareness is the aim of Authentic Movement.

Ground form

The ground form is the dyadic exchange between a mover and a witness. It is called the ground form because it constitutes the relational basis on which other Authentic Movement practice formats build and rely. In this format the mover allows any impulse to guide her through spontaneous sequences of movement and stillness. When time is called by the witness, the mover opens her eyes. There may be a quiet transition time, and then mover and witness will come together to speak with each other. Both participants use percept language. By example, the witness gradually teaches the mover how percept language is best used to relate experiences and witnessing. This dyadic format can constitute the primal relatedness between self and self, self and other, self and world, self and inner witness, mother and child, partners, friends or siblings.

Timing

Timing is important in Authentic Movement, and agreement of the length of practice elements prior to engagement is essential. Movement time can be from as little as 1 minute to up to an hour in long circles. Quite often, the time span is about 20 minutes movement time for an individual mover or a small group. Correct timekeeping is the responsibility of the witness as a mover's sense of time can become distorted when moving with her eyes closed. Movement time can feel stretched or compressed to the mover. The witness calls time with a bell or simply with her voice, asking the mover to end her movement and to open her eyes. Transition time can be adjusted to the need of the mover; it can be as long as or longer than the movement element. Verbal processing and witnessing time is often equal to or longer than the movement element. The witness/teacher is the time-keeper, safeguarding the mover's return to full waking consciousness. The timings of all elements of the practice are adjusted according to the material emerging in movement and verbal recall, in accordance with the capacity of all participants.

Transition

Transition is the time span between the movement, observed by the witness, and the subsequent sharing of experiences using language. As a rule of thumb, transition time is as long as the preceding movement time. It is a time to adjust to full waking consciousness and to allow semi-conscious experiences to take form in feelings, images, memories, thoughts and words, beginning a journey of integration and recognition. It is also a time for the witness to feel and remember what she has seen, to locate images and sensations within her own embodied self, and to begin to form thoughts and words in preparation for sharing with the mover. This time is silent. Transition can be used for a simple walk inside or outside of the studio or used for being quiet with nature if such is available. Transition time can also be a space for creative transpositions via visual art media that can provide a helpful reference point in the subsequent reflection between mover and witness. One of my students transposed her experience of strong sensations in her lower back into a perfectly formed, life-size vertebra using clay. Other visual expressions may be more expressive of emotions and feelings and use different materials. Writing during transition time can prepare the mover and the witness for speaking. Sometimes movers and witnesses read from such writings.

Invitation to speak

In Authentic Movement practice, the mover speaks first about their experience, recollecting significant or memorable moments. Second, the witness may be invited by the mover to share her witnessing. Sometimes the mover does not require or wish for any verbal witnessing by her witness. The witness respects this wish and holds her silence. Sometimes a simple acknowledgement of 'I see you' or 'I hear you' suffices as witnessing.

Remembering

Remembering is a fitting term as it makes literal reference to body-mind memory: re-membering or retracing members of the body. As the mover learns to draw a verbal map of her movement using percept language, she may also re-member by repeating certain gestures and movements, doing them again. The witness is careful not to simply mimick the mover's gestures. However, a gestural re-membering, when done sensitively and with permission by the mover, can create affirmative feedback.

Containment

When the witness is practising in the service of the mover, she endevours to contain what she has seen and felt during the movement. She only reflects back to the mover what she has heard the mover remember, even when she has also seen other movements and feelings unfold. There are other ways to practise, some of which are described in the guide, but this is the safest method to protect the mover from unwanted projections by the witness.

What can happen when the mover does not contain her impressions of what she has seen? She may tell the mover of her own feelings, for example 'a great sadness' she experienced when she was watching the mover. The mover doesn't remember this about herself but doesn't want to contradict her witness. However, she may feel disturbed in her own truth and wonder: was she perhaps not conscious of feeling sad? She may also feel that she has not been seen and heard in her experiences, and as a consequence she may feel isolated and even unsafe. She may close up and manifest a containment that her witness did not offer her. The witness may not notice this. The contact and intimacy that might have been possible between the two has taken a step back. An opportunity for being seen and being heard has been missed.

Languaging

The word languaging is sometimes used to describe the particular process of finding words to describe movement and witnessing experiences in Authentic Movement. The term 'languaging' was coined by M. Swain in a different context to describe a language learner's efforts to speak meaningfully in a foreign tongue. Swain found that the mind has to consciously focus when speaking a second language and that this effort turns speaking into a conscious act (Swain 1985). The term is differently used in contemporary discourses in the humanities, where it describes using language fluidly and experimentally. This is an attempt to dispose of a language of oppression, colonialism and patriarchy. Languaging in this context makes up new and sometimes poetic and incomplete ways of speaking and abandons clear grammatical rules. Both this and Swain's use of the word contain aspects of its use in Authentic Movement.

Languaging in Authentic Movement can be seen as similar to Swain's notion of having to make a conscious effort. Learners in Authentic Movement wrangle with finding the correct words to describe their movement and meanings. Authentic Movement is "a study of articulation not only of body but of word" (Adler 2002, p. 16). Languaging enables the emergence of an embodied consciousness. Unfortunately in many adaptations of Authentic Movement, both in and out of dance therapy, taking conscious time to language is forgotten. Yet, considered languaging makes a profound difference to movers' and witnesses' perceptions of themselves and others. Authentic Movement practiced without knowledge of its languaging part lacks its most useful pedagogical and therapeutic tool.

Percept language

The use of silence and language between a mover and a witness plays an essential role in Authentic Movement practice and is paramount to its integrity and directly related to the value that may be derived from it. At times mover and witness hold silence in order to practice containment of the moved and witnessed materials. When language is used to recall and relate the movement experiences it is in a very specific form: percept language. The skills of percept language were adapted by Adler and originate in the work of John and Joyce Weir. Adler relates this at the beginning of her primer (2002) and in an interview with Tina Stromsted and Neala Haze:

> John Weir had also taught participants "percept language", in which individuals are asked to own their own experience using the words "I saw..." or "I felt..." rather than projecting or interpreting or judging other people's experiences.
>
> (Haze & Stromsted 2007, p. 114)

Percept language trains learners to own their experiences by using the present tense in these I-statements. Movement and witnessing become present when spoken in that way. 'I saw' becomes 'I see' and 'I felt' becomes 'I feel'. The present tense relates events that lie in the past but that are brought into the present moment by the speaker, reliving them at that moment.

> Our frame of reference for the lab, then, is that each of us is continually perceiving and organising his world in his unique way, never precisely the same as anyone else. I am "doing" myself and you are "doing" yourself. Your "existence" is for me always my perception of you, the "you-in-me", and I "exist" for you only as the "me-in-you". You are there, you act, you may even physically influence me. This has the consequence of changing the "you-in-me" and the "me-in-you". How I "do" the "you-in-me" is determined by my needs, my perceptions, and my past experiences.
>
> (Weir 1975, p. 9)

In other words, each one of us has our own perceptions and perspectives on what is perceived. We each see, hear and experience the world in our own unique way. Importantly, this frame of reference includes other persons and so strongly influences our relationships. By realising that my own experience is always my own, and by stating so, I can allow another person's reality to coexist. This permission to be different creates a clearing in which relationship can take place. This solipsistic philosophy of perception of self and other is embodied in Authentic Movement by the performative situation of a mover and witness within the present moment. It is continued in the use of percept language in the recall between mover and witness.

It is, I am, always my own responsibility. This is true both for how I do myself and how you do yourself. We conclude that the perceptual elements of our interpersonal interactions consist of a 'you', a 'me', a 'you-in-me' and a 'me-in-you'.

(Weir 1975, p. 9)

The linguistic tool of stating this insight, translating it into a way of speaking with the other, enables speakers to take full responsibility for the content and effect of their spoken words. What is spoken is theirs through and through and the recipient of their statement is empowered to agree or to disagree from their own perception and perspective. By creating this understanding a clear separation of I and Thou is made. This is not to keep apart but to foster a coming together as a new intimate sharing of two individuals that is neither based in agreement nor in disagreement but in the capacity to acknowledge the other.

There is no abdication to others as in the use of 'they', no generalisation as in the use of 'one', no corroboration as in the use of 'we', no projection or objectification as in the use of 'you', no reminiscing as in the use of the past tense, no longing as in the use of the future tense, and no correction or wishing, as in the use of a conjunctive. Further, there is no object. Instead, there is a first-person, singular, the 'I', that stands responsible for her perceptions in the present moment. Stromsted states that "These 'I' statements later became the cornerstone of Adler's teaching of the role of the witness" (Stromsted 2007b, p. 247). Used in Authentic Movement practices, percept language follows a methodological and epistemological solipsism, where the subject states that perceptions of the external world depend upon the internal world of the individual speaking. Mix (2006) remarks that whilst Weir's invention of percept language has positively impacted many private and professional lives, it has received little credit in the literature (outside of Adler's Discipline of Authentic Movement).

The context of this new percept language in Authentic Movement is also its rationale: the mover makes herself open and vulnerable in disclosing herself in movement, gesture and word to a witness. She empowers herself by owning her experiences. Any words (and gestures) that are uttered in response have to mirror an equally self-responsible owning. These words or any silence need to convey full regard and respect for her perceptions and integrity. Witnessing in Authentic Movement is a discipline, according to Adler's teachings, not a mere account, less yet a narrative, a tale and definitely not an outpouring. A safe psychological space in Authentic Movement is one where the spoken word is used in the described disciplined manner.

Many times, everyday language is used in Authentic Movement practice. Understandably this is the first and spontaneous way in which to process and share some of the extraordinary, profound and sometimes overwhelming experiences of Authentic Movement. However, the movement experience is only half of the story. Without the relatively strict rules of percept language much projection, confusion and disappointment can result in the verbal witnessing process. Practitioners are well-advised to study and learn percept language. It will be worth it.

Affirmation

In Authentic Movement practice, also an affirmative language is used between mover and witness. Statements in percept language, such as 'I hear you' and 'I see you', affirm shared moments in a simple, matter-of-fact way. When felt and spoken in the first person and present time (see also percept language) this factual simplicity can touch the other person deeply and, as Adler has stated, fulfil a deep cultural longing by the individual to be seen and heard.

Affirmative statements can also fulfil the speaker's need to speak, to be heard and to share by using reliable, true words.

> I discover my uniqueness by taking ownership of myself and my experience, and by assuming responsibility for my behavior. I cannot compete with you, or anyone else in this process. I, and only I can "do" me in my own way. Moving always at my own pace, there can be no win-lose. I am what I am, when I am.
>
> (Weir 1975, p. 12)

This affirmative statement is also a premise of Authentic Movement. It can be held in mind and spoken as it serves as a reminder to participants of this unique premise underlying the practice.

Another example of affirmation, this time communicated by eye contact and gesture, is the so-called 'sprouting', a humorous term invented, according to my personal memory, during a long and tiring circle in one of Adler's Italian retreats. The sprouting of witnesses may be initiated by a witness in a long circle who feels that her own and/or others' witnessing is waning. It is a call for support between witnesses to maintain wakeful attention and consciousness in what can be a tiring task. Making eye contact and reaching out sideways with her arms she seeks to connect with other witnesses in the circle, who will affirm her by echoing her movement, altogether creating a gestural circle around the movers' space and acknowledging their being present.

Moving witness

Moving witness is a development of the ground form by introducing a second mover to the dyad of one mover and one witness. Two movers move at the same time with their eyes closed in front of one teacher/witness. As in the ground form, they follow their own inner impulses for movement, but now they must be also aware of the other mover in the space. Their witness has to widen her attention to encompass both movers. This formation of three creates a more complex field of external stimuli and internal responses in both the movers and the witness. In the movers a shift from being 'the only one' to 'being with another' takes place. In effect, each mover now also becomes a meta-witness to the other mover although 'blindly'. They each sense, hear and energetically feel the other mover's journey and actions. These perceptions become a rich new source for each mover. Yet, as before, each mover's experiences are considered and processed as pertaining to herself, not as information about the other mover.

The desire to 'tell all' between the two movers can be strong. If not contained within silence and percept language, conversations following moving can become narratives eager to establish common meeting points. It is not the learning purpose of this practice format to find shared territory. Instead, its aim is to add complexity to experiences, simulating a more real life situation. Much discipline is required at this stage, especially when the format widens even further to allow more movers to move all at the same time forming a group. To be recognised by a fellow mover can be special and profound but the aim of this practice is to learn about oneself. Shared experiences can easily become projections and it is an art to hold these within. To wait until the other mover speaks of her own perceptions and to see if there really was meeting point means that the subtlety and intimacy when encountered can be greater.

Silent witness

The silent witness is a development of practicing the moving witness. It means to witness visually by the side of an experienced witness but to practice strict containment of one's desire to verbally share what one has seen. A new witness is a silent witness for some time and this practice element protects other movers from hearing spoken statements which may be unwanted or can't as yet be phrased in percept language. It protects the mover from projections and judgements which can be confusing and hurtful. A silent witness learns to contain what she sees and, instead of sharing with the mover, she only writes down her experiences and speaks together with the teacher/witness. This way the new witness can safely learn that whatever she sees and experiences is her own material, her imagination and her feelings. She learns to honour the freedom of a mover to be in a safe atmosphere of accepting silence. It does not mean that the silent witness cannot make eye contact, in fact, her alert silent presence is enhanced by this simple and powerful form of communication. The moving witness and the silent witness can be combined in one role, whereby the silent witness simply does not speak after her movement but just pertains to listening to the speakers and paying attention to her own sensations, feelings and images at the same time.

Speaking witness

In this phase of learning, a practised silent witness begins to speak with a mover. Initially, as in psychotherapeutic applications of the practice, the witness will ask the mover for permission to speak and if granted, reflects back what she has heard the mover say about her movement. To do so she may begin sentences with 'I hear you', making reference to the mover's verbal statements. Later in the learning process, in peer and in group formats, the witness may be invited by the mover to also recall the movement in her own words. Still the witness will only relate what has also been related by the mover, and using such percept language statements as to make clear that her memories of the movement are her own. This becomes particularly important when she first maps out a kinaesthetic map of movement and adds feeling, images and intuitions. To help clarity, speaking witnesses always name themselves in their present tense statements, i.e. 'I see; I hear; I sense; I feel', thus stating that their perceptions belong to none other than themselves. Through the committed practice of moving and witnessing in this style of speaking, the capacity to see oneself and another with increasing understanding, precision and empathy develop. In collective body formats speaking may take on a less direct form. The circle of movers is addressed rather than an individual, but the seen is always related as pertaining to the individual speaker's experience. There are many subtle practice stages that a speaking witness will go through to develop her skills and these are best guided by an experienced teacher.

Collective body

Collective body is a practice format in which movers and witnesses work together in a group. This usually only takes place when movers have developed the capacity to remember and recall movement, and are capable of containing and speaking observations. In collective body, participants learn to move together and speak together as a whole group on a level playing field. The concept of collective body suggests a deep connectedness between all participants on a spatial, kinaesthetic, emotional, cellular and energetic level. Surrendering to such a notion of group and moving can feel like being part of a larger, collective body. Clear individual consciousness is required to allow safe entry to and exit from such events, particularly when the group's collective needs drive unforeseeable movement configurations and sound expressions. Collective body work embraces the notion of the post-human and can be used in developing new understandings in groups, societies and ecologies. Collective body work can enable journeys beyond the becoming of individual embodiment and in favour of becoming a collective belonging. Shared habitats (Goldhahn 2007) can emerge.

Long circle

Long circle is a practice format for experienced movers and witnesses. Here all participants are simultaneously potential witnesses and movers. Witnesses can respond spontaneously to the collective body by becoming movers and decide for themselves when to return to their place in the circle to, again, witness the group. Each mover, in pursuit of their own pathway and movement, is also open to the collective impressions of sound and movement and their own contributions in turn shape an overall evolution of the group. Participants can experience themselves as active members of a constantly evolving collective body. Collective dramas, such as loss, grief, delight and celebration, are enacted without any visual orientation and can appear like spontaneous 'choreographies'. Each participant constructs their own meanings of these 'blind performances'. Interrelationships and synchronicities can be discovered as being permeating and profound.

Breathing circle

In breathing circle, participants divide into two equal groups of movers and witnesses and take turns in moving and witnessing. The space within the circle of witnesses is their movement space. The length of movement time is agreed. Likened to a breath in and a breath out, participants take turns observing and moving in equal intervals of time. They move in and out of the circle transiting from seeing to closing their eyes and back again. Breathing circles require advanced skills to transit seamlessly from mover consciousness to witness consciousness and an ability to contain experiences until it is time to gather and speak at the end of one or several rounds of breathing circle.

Speaking circle

After group formats such as breathing circle and long circle, speaking circles are formed. Participants take it in turns to speak about their own experiences of moving as part of the group. Spoken witnessing may be offered in turn. In experienced circles verbal witnessing may no longer be given in sole service of an individual mover but in service of the collective. This type of witnessing is sometimes spoken intuitively, impersonally, without naming or addressing an individual mover. Speaking circles share experiences in a ritualised form of percept language where, sometimes, profound new insights can emerge through a freer, poetic form of languaging and echoing others' statements or gestures. The intricacy of rules that a particular peer group might want to adhere to gives much scope to reflect timing and readiness. The important aspect is, again, to safeguard individual needs within a collective. On the whole, the use of percept language is the most useful and safest way to engage in speaking circles.

In collective group formats, separate moving and speaking circles can aid the study of containment, protection and the learning of percept language. After a breathing circle, witnesses and movers can form separate circles to speak in percept language. In those separate circles movers are not named but referred to simply as 'the mover who...', thereby explicitly respecting the privacy of each individual mover (see also Silent witness).

Echoing

Echoing is another element in Authentic Movement speaking practice. Participants repeat a phrase another speaker has made and that they feel particularly attuned to. Within speaking circles, this can be done individually by different speakers in turn or in unison together by several members of a speaking circle at once. Echoing is an affirmative ritual for both the individual and the group. Shared experience, empathy and collectivity are evoked and made present. For example, a mover's statement might be: 'I rise up on my toes and stretch my whole body upwards. My whole face smiles. I feel delight.' She may be echoed by her witness saying: 'I feel delight.' or 'My whole face smiles.' or, simply, 'I rise up on my toes and stretch'; depending on what the witness saw and felt in the mover's movement or what she heard and particularly empathised with when she heard the mover speak.

Conscious body

A conscious body is a mystical concept (Adler 2002) and, for most Western bodies and minds, an unattainable goal. Human consciousness can very rarely be absolute and may be considered to be utopian. However, the concept of a conscious body, when considered with due circumspection, may be glimpsed at times of deep and moving insight into bodily knowledge.

Psychological dangers

Authentic Movement practices should not be simply experimented with without having a profound understanding of the body and psyche and of ethical and safe boundaries. Authentic Movement practice can enhance and develop the integrity of the individual and this has to be done carefully with reverence to the unconscious mind that is invoked. Involuntary altered states of consciousness and/or psychosis are contraindications. Instead individuals will benefit from somatic work and dance therapy designed to ground the psyche within the kinaesthetic and haptic reality of the body. People with a history of experiencing hallucinations, drug abuse or self-harm must be advised against practising with closed eyes in a wakeful state, as this can trigger phosphenes and a recurrence of unwanted symptoms.

Any too lighthearted or uninformed approach to the unconscious and to Authentic Movement can be dangerous and yield unwanted results, such as confused states of mind or serious, and even irretrievable psychosis at worst. In my view, and shared with many other dance therapists, psychotherapists and teachers of the Discipline of Authentic Movement (Adler 2002) this is to be safeguarded against. A trained and trusted guide must be sought in all these matters as the unconscious, when encountered unprepared, can be like a labyrinth that one may not find one's way out again. Authentic Movement can be deep, powerful and an entry into deep unconsciously held material. It is the entry and exit from such places and the timing and spacing of such encounters that have to be very carefully prepared and held by an experienced psychotherapist and trainer. As Elliot recalls:

> I experienced two people on two separate occasions go into an acute psychotic break during an Authentic Movement workshop. This was not a class, it was an introductory workshop.
>
> (Elliott 2021)

I recommend *The dancing body in psychotherapy: Reflections on Somatic psychotherapy and Authentic Movement* (Stromsted 2007a) for understanding the distinct use of Authentic Movement in psychotherapy and for a somatic assessment for the purposes of safety.

Consciousness and unconsciousness

The declared aim of Authentic Movement is to become more embodied and more conscious. This is practised by getting to know, experience and language the unconscious. There is no absolute of either qualities and this is an important point, similar to my questions about the notion of "authenticity". There is no absolute boundary, rather consciousness and unconscious are fluid states that each takes from and exchanges with the other, they are littoral realms with no fixed boundaries.

Boredom can occur in Authentic Movement as in psychoanalytic practices. Both the witness and the mover may become bored. This can have many reasons, for example avoidance, and can result in sleepy, non-witnessing unconsciousness. Also, the actual process of decolonisation of the body-mind can produce sleepiness and boredom. In any case, there is no judgement in

Authentic Movement about boredom and, when it occurs, it can be explored in percept language.

Practicing online

Geopolitical and economic reasons have prompted many practitioners to offer online work. Unfortunately it remains a poor substitute for the privilege of being in the presence of another person. It is presence that online 'presence' seeks to imitate, and digital innovations, 3D projections and holograms all have just that one aim: to bridge the physical distance and to emulate what cannot be had for real. Recent research (Bailenson 2021) has shown that the close proximity of participants to their respective screens produces an intimacy that is inappropriate for most social encounters. Being seen digitally so close up does not create greater intimacy with another mover or witness, it rather distorts the actual relationship. Being deceptively close to another mover or witness cannot ameliorate the fact that we are far apart physically and have to work very hard to create a sense of intimacy. Authentic Movement is not entirely satisfactory in online, screen-based work. As the virtual is employed in order to be seen moving, the potential of intimacy can be foreclosed. Mover and witness remain outside of each others presence and physical reach. Technology tries to emulate presence, but it is not presence. Online sessions can be very hard work for participants as even higher than usual levels of awareness and imagination are required to fill the interpersonal gap. To hold in mind the complexities of being close and far away all at the same time is demanding and can distract from the original purpose (see also Chapter 11 of this volume).

Moving outdoors

Outdoor practice usually lacks the clear containment that a studio space provides. However, if participants have attained mover and witness consciousness, moving outdoors can add stimulation and enrichment and be sought for very specific explorations and responses to environmental factors. These can include encounters with non- or post-human movers and imagined witnesses such as architecture, trees, plants, animals, rocks and water. I would suggest that moving outdoors requires prior experience indoors and the application of a very specific aspect of Authentic Movement practices. See also Chapter 12 of this volume.

Level playing field

Level playing field means the equality and parity of all participants, whether that is in dyadic encounters of a single witness and mover or in collective body work. Each individual's viewpoint, which is always their own, is honoured and respected as belonging and being valid to that individual. Unfortunately the high cost and limited availability to study Authentic Movement largely restricts access to the white, educated middle classes. Young people, people of colour, men and people with different gender identities can seem to have less direct access to Authentic Movement. Whilst a level playing field is inherent, to come to and access Authentic Movement in the first place is not always easy. I would like to see it more widely available to different communities and to be less expensive. Sponsored community groups could be set up around experienced teachers to train and distribute the practices into society where they could do much good to raise embodied consciousness in the knowledge that we are all equal.

Some misconceptions

The umbrella term Authentic Movement is used by many practitioners/teachers who don't specifically follow Adler's Discipline of Authentic Movement but may use some elements thereof. It is useful for students to establish what background and tradition a teacher follows and which, if any, of the concepts described in this guide are included in their teaching. Authentic Movement practice in its most basic form, i.e. non-directive, 'blind' movement followed by speaking between a mover and a witness, is now used by many improvisers within dance therapy, dance, performance, choreography and in popular, very large group forms of 'ecstatic dance' such as Gabrielle Roth's 5 Rhythms. It is unfortunate when in many of those contexts the parameters and practices designed to foster and develop safety, personal development and consciousness are little known or not applied. Thus some perilous paths open up: in the best case scenario the practice becomes shallow, participants cannot experience the depth of embodiment that they are longing for. In this case, the practice loses its potential power, but mover and witness remain relatively safe. In another scenario the practice becomes unsafe, participants become confused or disturbed. For example, when only a few safety rules are met, participants can and do get hurt. When permissive touch is given free reign participants will find it difficult to know their own boundaries. There are many misconceptions for example that the practice is 'very easy'. In my supervision of postgraduate students of dance therapy I have come across frequent statements similar to: 'Yes, we have done authentic movement in class. It seemed so easy. You do it so differently. There is so much more to it, so much more to learn that I didn't know was Authentic Movement'.

Tiredness

Authentic Movement practices demand a high level of focus. Moving and witnessing for longer than attention span allows can lead to inattentive practice.

Whilst boredom can be part of the MoverWitness psychosomatic dynamic, plain tiredness can place the mover into an unheld space, leaving them feeling unseen. These are opposite outcomes of what the practice aims to achieve.

Music and sound

Music is not necessary nor desirable. It is not part of the tradition and roots of this practice and does not belong to a space in which a mover experiences being seen by another in their search for their very own being in movement. As Elliott states: "I believe the Form has become appropriated like much in the dance world, people have taken Authentic Movement and changed it. People put on relaxing music or any kind of music for that matter and invite people to close their eyes" (Elliott 2021). Sound and soundings generated by movers themselves are a different matter. They can be important expressions that accompany movement and contribute to a powerful soundscape. It is a matter for participants to agree to what extent they wish to include or exclude sound as auditory perceptions and sensitivities vary greatly. A silent practice of movement is Authentic Movement's first premise and is easier to concentrate on. Sound adds another layer of experience and can be a distraction or an enrichment. This has to be considered in each individual case.

Group size

In safe Authentic Movement practice, group size matters and is in direct relationship to the inner capacity of participants and the teacher/witness. The dyadic ground form is always recommended for beginners. My own training with Adler took place in a group of about twenty women, but in my own teaching, I like a group size of eight to twelve participants.

References

Adler, J. (1987). Who is the witness, a description of Authentic Movement. *Contact Quarterly*, 12, no 1, 1987, (pp. 20–29).

Adler, J. (2002). *Offering from the conscious body: the Discipline of Authentic Movement*. Inner Traditions, Rochester, Vermont.

Adler, J. (2019). Somatics Festival 2019, *A.P.E.@ Hawley and The School For Contemporary Dance & Thought with Historic Northampton, Northampton Open Media, and the Smith College Department of Dance, 19–23 September 2019*.

Bailenson, J. N. (2021). Nonverbal Overload: A Theoretical Argument for the Causes of Zoom Fatigue. *Technology, Mind, and Behavior, 2 (1)*.

Ehrenberg, S. & Wood. K. (2011). Kinaesthetic empathy: concepts and contexts. *Dance Research Journal*, Volume 43, (2), (pp. 113–118).

Elliott, W. (2021). Email to Eila Goldhahn, 7 March 2021.

Goldhahn, E. (2007). *Shared habitats, the MoverWitness paradigm.* [Doctoral dissertation, Dartington College of Arts and of Plymouth, UK].

Goldhahn, E. (2010a). The MoverWitness exchange: interdisciplinary pedagogy and communication tool, towards an embodied and empathetic laboratory. Conference proceedings. *Kinesthetic Empathy: Concepts and Contexts,* The Watching Dance Project, Manchester University (22–23 April, 2010).

Haze, N. & Stromsted, T. (1994). An interview with Jant Adler. In Pallaro, P. (ed.) (1999). *Authentic Movement: essays by Mary Starks Whitehouse, Janet Adler and Joan Chodorow.* Jessica Kingsley, London & Philadelphia.

Lotringer, S. & Virilio, P. (2005). *The accident of art.* MIT Press/Semiotext, Cambridge, Mass.

Mix, P. J. (2006). A monumental legacy: the unique and unheralded contributions of John and Joyce Weir to the human development field. *The Journal of Applied Behavioural Sciences,* Volume 42, No. 3, (pp. 276–299).

Pallaro, P. (ed.) (1999). *Authentic Movement: essays by Mary Starks-Whitehouse, Janet Adler and Joan Chodorow.* Jessica Kingsley, London and Philadelphia.

Pallaro, P. (ed.) (2007). *Authentic Movement, moving the body, moving the self, being moved.* A collection of essays, Vol 2. Jessica Kingsley, London.

Sheets-Johnstone, M. (2019). The silence of movement, a beginning empirical phenomenological exposition of the powers of a corporeal semiotics. *The American Journal of Semiotics,* 35.1–2 (2019), (pp. 33–54).

Stromsted, T. (2007a). The dancing body in psychotherapy: Reflections on Somatic psychotherapy and Authentic Movement. Pallaro, P. (ed.) (2007) *Authentic Movement, moving the body, moving the self, being moved: a collection of essays, Vol 2.* Jessica Kingsley, London, (pp. 202–220).

Stromsted, T. (2007b). The Discipline of Authentic Movement as mystical practice: evolving moments in Janet Adler's life and work. Pallaro, P. (ed.) (2007) *Authentic Movement, moving the body, moving the self, being moved: a collection of essays, Vol 2.* Jessica Kingsley, London, (pp. 244–259).

Swain, M. (1985). Communicative competence: some roles of comprehensible input and comprehensible output in its development. *Input in second language acquisition.* Gass, S. & Madden, C. (Eds.) Newbury House, Rowley, MA. (pp. 235–253).

Weir, J. (1975). The personal growth laboratory: The Laboratory Method of Changing and Learning: Theory and Application. *Science and behaviour books.* K. Benne, L.P. Bradford, J.R. Gibb, R.D. Lippitt (eds.), Palo Alto, California.

Part II

The art of the MoverWitness

Chapter 4

Visualising movers and witnesses

Introduction

This chapter is based on an essay first published in the journal E-motion of The Association for Dance Movement Psychotherapy UK in 2009.

Whilst Authentic Movement is related to the art form of dance, as in moving, the practice has deeply embedded visual aspects. These are manifest in witnessing. The witness has her eyes open to see whilst the mover closes her eyes to listen inward. Whilst witnessing has many other levels of perception, its visual sense is the dominant one.

The combination of these two aspects, moving and witnessing, in this live ritual situates the practice within the field of performance, it is a performative event. Yet performance is mostly associated with a public event. With a few exceptions, for example in community long circles as developed by Sperry and Tsetse (2003, 2007), Authentic Movement is practised in a safe and private space. This nourishes creative and empathetic processes in the confidentiality of trusted one-to-one or group exchanges. In my role as a teacher of Authentic Movement, I respect these protected spaces. However, as an arts-led researcher, I want to find ways in which I can investigate and communicate aesthetic aspects of Authentic Movement that are most meaningful to me and that I feel could speak to a public audience too.

The philosopher Hannah Arendt states, there is a need to deprivatise and deindividualise certain inner and private experiences. This is a political act.

> Compared with the reality which comes from being seen and heard, even the greatest forces of intimate life – the passions of the heart, the thoughts of the mind, the delights of the senses – lead an uncertain, shadowy kind of existence unless and until they are transformed, deprivatised and deindividualised, as it were, into a shape to fit them for public appearance.
>
> (Arendt 1958, p. 50)

Confronting the dilemma of Authentic Movement's privacy and how I, as a mover or a witness, would feel in the presence of a public, I decided to develop my arts-led research using film and visual art, instead of live performance.

DOI: 10.4324/9781003222309-6

Visualisations

Visualisations using art materials are commonly used in Authentic Movement's so-called transition time, when participants process and express movement and witness experiences prior to speaking with each other. During the reflective dialogue it is usual for movers and witnesses to use visual imagery to relate their respective experiences. This may be sharing visualisations produced during transition time or a verbal recall of visual impressions. Visuality relates easily and directly to the imagination and the heart. On the most simple yet profound level the mover asks: 'Am I seen?' and the witness may answer: 'I see you'. But visuality can also describe other levels of perception. Whilst Authentic Movement engages all the different senses, feelings and intuitions, the visual sense being culturally the most dominant one is most commonly reflected in Authentic Movement's language. It is this fascinating intersection between movement, visuality and language that inspired me to use art media to explore Authentic Movement's workings.

Shaun McNiff's view that making visual art is an appropriate and powerful tool for the investigation of another arts practice was encouraging (McNiff 1998). Dance therapy has tended to sideline creative arts as valid research methods in its own field, favouring empirical studies instead. By doing so dance therapy has understandably strengthened its battle for recognition within the health professions. Scientific research methodologies are often employed and believed to best prove the therapy's effectiveness as a treatment (Berrol 2000). Yet by doing so, these methodologies can sideline dance therapy's inherent and powerful artistic, anthropological and cultural roots. The aesthetic relevance of dance and movement as an art form in therapy can thus play a secondary role in many studies. Using the arts as a primary tool in research, I wanted to affirm that dance and movement belong to the family of the arts and have unique knowledge to impart.

After some initial experimenting together with dancers and a camera, I determined that throughout my research process I would maintain the ethical framework as learned in my studies with Adler. I found this framework to be closely compliant with academic research ethics standards in the arts and humanities.

Another motivation for my arts-led research was my wish to communicate Authentic Movement's workings and aesthetics with a wider public than it normally reaches. I wanted to share some of its strong visual qualities and give an insight into ordinary people, not necessarily dancers, moving with integrity, conveying beauty and meaning. Introducing an interdisciplinary dialogue between two art forms, dance movement and visual arts, enabled me to experiment with Authentic Movement's transferability. This way my question of whether the methods of Authentic Movement could perhaps be applied as a research method was tested. For example, in writing and talking about visual art I used percept language to name different parts of my experience. The arts-led research community at Dartington College of Arts offered many opportunities and challenges for my project; researchers were concerned with contemporary theories and performative arts in their many facets, and less so in psychotherapy or mysticism, important aspects in Adler's work. I chose to site my PhD research in this particular setting as it enabled me to return to the roots of my artistic training and beliefs. Here, I hoped to develop a new focus in Authentic Movement; one focused on its art, its creativity and its ethics.

In the reflective writing for my thesis, I described the various layers of my practices of moving, witnessing and making visual art with reference to my own embodied knowledge, closely mirroring the practice of languaging. When reflecting the complex relationships between the moved, the visualised, the witnessed and the spoken, my written texts progressed. With each turn of phrase and new paragraph, I braided another small aspect of the practice's transient complexity into my writing, endeavouring to reach ever closer to its essence. Whilst unwrapping the practice's embodied reality into a linear dimension of sentences was useful, writing also revealed its inherent limitations of disclosing an ephemeral, living practice. However, the difficulties associated with expressing the fleeting nature of movement, observation and ritual solely through the written word seemed to indicate a different creative route.

I realised that my subject matter required a treatment that mirrored the embodied, performative and visual elements of Authentic Movement practices. By engaging my research questions with processes of creating art, I found that my artistic image-making became a potent visual tool to ask questions, to gain new and complex insights, and to share these with others. Many artworks emerged from my engagement with visual media. Sometimes I was reminded of an arts therapeutic process in which a client given the opportunity to express herself produces a swell of creative output. As with my research writing before, my visual art-making became first prolific and then more selective and refined.

Film was an obvious medium through which I could apply my witnessing skills to filming Authentic Movement in action. I applied a singular, still perspective, following the subject in a quiet and meditative way from where I was seated. Participants in my film projects were asked for consent prior to and also after filming. They were invited to view and vet my filmed material and to then decide whether to give their consent for its further use in my arts-led research and associated public showings. With their valuable contributions, I created a series of films, installations and paintings. I called my filming camera-witnessing (Goldhahn 2007) because I transferred one of Authentic Movement's cornerstones, witnessing, to another medium, the lens-based, digital seeing and recording. Some of my films of Authentic Movement can be accessed via www.sharedhabitat.net.

From these digital documents, I chose some still images. I looked for those moments when, as a witness, I had felt particularly alerted and connected to a mover, when perhaps a moment of kinaesthetic empathy (Ehrenberg & Wood 2011; Foster 2011) had taken place or when a memory, feeling or image had been evoked within me. I was interested to see how and if these moments would manifest in a still image taken out of the context of the film and whether such an image could, in turn, communicate with a public audience. Some images passed this requirement whilst others did not reach the bar. One particular digital image that met with my expectation, I titled *The Wall*. This image depicts the moment when a mover touches the surface of a wall with his hands, arms and thoracic torso in an intensely haptic experience in which his proprioceptive senses are visibly alert. In his self-reflection the mover spoke of encountering the wall as if touching such a surface for the first time. This was a sensual and nonverbal experience. As a witness I felt closely drawn into this particular moment. Building up a painting on canvas with layers on top of the original digital image, the depth I remembered the movement moment evoked in me, finally re-emerged. By painting the mover and 'his' wall complete with electrical sockets and a faint fall of light from above, I am reminded of an intensely shared moment between the mover and myself as his witness. It became significant and meaningful to me and I wanted to share this experience with others as it points to the unique potential of kinaesthetic empathy in Authentic Movement. The painting created on top of a digital image on canvas visualises the complex interplay of surface and depth of field that can occur in a witness's experience, something that the digital image alone could not do. A mover can seem very near to or far away from a witness, not just by merit of their actual distance but by merit of the inner engagement of the witness with the mover. The painting plays artistically with the rapture of a shared moment. It does not represent well in black and white print, but it can be viewed digitally at www.sharedhabitat.net.

Another image that has captured this sense of enrapture by a mover for me as a witness, was a portrait of a mover who also kindly allowed me to use her image. This image is initially perceived as a painting but it is actually a small size print of a film still. Two images show her fine physiognomy display a subtle yet very moving change within her facial features; feelings were expressed and the camera-witnessed images communicate the mover's and witness's shared experience of these moments, again this too can be accessed via www.sharedhabitat.net.

Other art films made together with dancer Malaika Sarco-Thomas also resulted in stills and paintings. There are three examples of the series *Malaika Dancing* included in this book as illustrations of this work. There are two small images below (Figure 4.1) and another larger one, that has been transformed into a painting, in Part III of this book (Figure 8.1, *Holding Hands*).

Adler's notion of a collective body (Adler 2002) can produce a sense of equality and belonging between movers and witnesses. Depending on the number of movers, an extremely complex pattern of movement and interactions can emerge which can be difficult to recall and process in language. This is explored in the next chapter, that explores and contextualises the witnessing and filming of a long circle, one of the formats in Authentic Movement, that can embue participants with a strong sense of collective belonging.

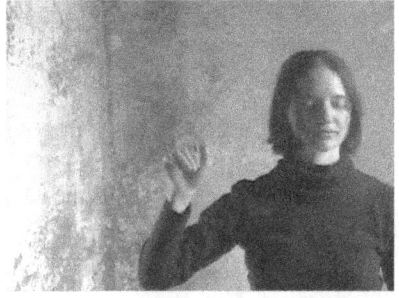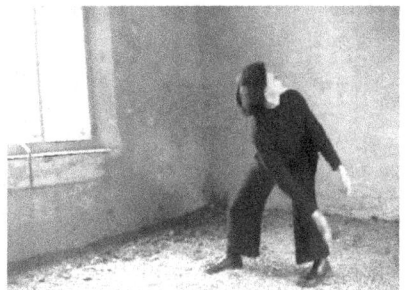

Figure 4.1 Two images of Malaika Dancing, film stills. Artist: Eila Goldhahn, 2005.

An exploration with textual, sculptural media arose out of my interest in notions of belonging. My works in the series *Shadows of our Former Selves* (Figure 4.2) explore belonging using very tangible haptic materials rather than lens-based, digital work. Starting with a well-known practice from dance therapy, I created cutouts of movers' body shapes.

> In the context of Movement Psychotherapy, I have regularly used a similar exercise but using paper and crayons. When a client's body image is diffuse and unclear this is a useful intervention to help him/her appreciate in a very concrete form what their body's physical size and shape is. Once the outline has been drawn on paper on the floor, clients fill it in. They name, colour and recreate their bodies through drawing, painting and writing on the different body parts. As therapeutic sessions progress and movement experience provides new understanding of clients' bodies and selves, the cutouts provide a map of the developing sense of a physically embodied, less alienated body image.
>
> (Goldhahn 2007)

Employing a similar starting point here in my art-making and exploring connectivity between bodies rather than an individual body, I drew around the silhouettes of two dancers in direct contact with each other lying on the floor. I then cut this interconnected shape out of an existing hide rug. Using this material instead of paper and crayons I created a completely different result and reading. There was no need to fill in and colour in because the medium itself was already full; full of texture and colour, full of previous uses, and full of the stories of other lives.

I had experienced my body in the actions of painting with the flow and colour of paint and crayon on canvas, for example when creating *The Wall.* Moving and making with textured materials, such as the hide, opened up a new haptic and proprioceptive field. The hide is tough and it requires effort to cut new shapes. Working with large scissors and kneeling on the floor,

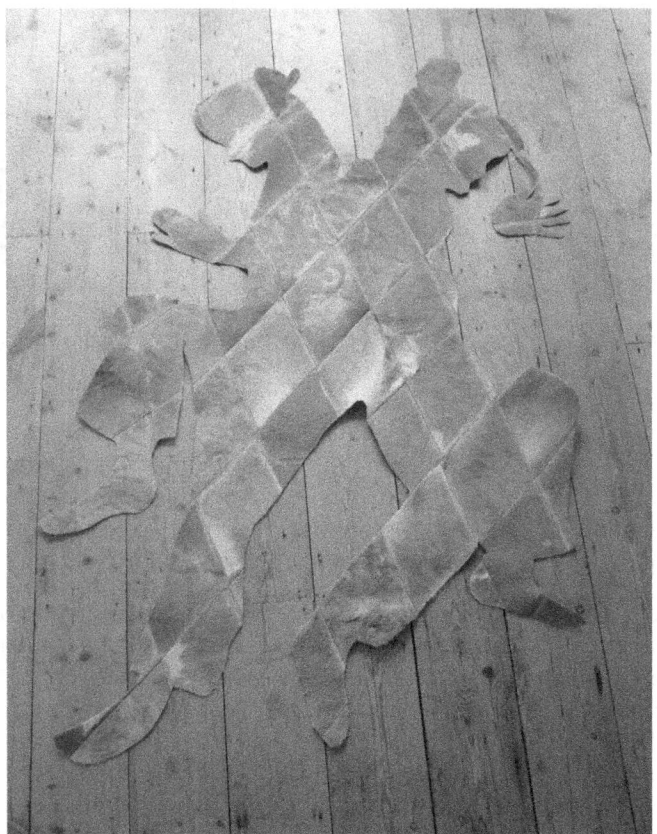

Figure 4.2 Shadows of our Former Selves, textile sculpture reusing deer hide.
Artist: Eila Goldhahn, 2006.

the making required intensity of effort within my right hand and arm and within my other limbs and torso to maintain balance within the correct position to execute the work. I found it curious how my physical position seemed to mirror that of an animal on all fours or perhaps a prehistoric hunter-gatherer cutting and cleaning hides; the materiality determined my body in movement.

Shadows of our Former Selves makes a more complex artistic statement than I initially anticipated. The fur-covered bodies can be read to relate to early developmental states when an embryo's body is covered in fine hairs. Also, the depicted body shapes, relaxed yet in movement, are reminiscent of developmental movement patterns in the floating medium of the womb. On another level, the work relates to interspecies' shared habitats, to ecology and to philosophies that bind together humans and animals as belonging together and of coming from the same family (Deleuze and Guattari 2004; Atterton & Calarco 2004). I hoped that this work could evoke associations of ecological implications for a new collective body, a collective body that could embrace not just humankind but animals, plants and nature at large. The use of the name shadow, also references Jung's notion of humans' unconscious nature, the collective shadow. The sculptures' only slightly raised flatness make them suitable both for floor and wall displays, with verticality or horizontality lending different readings. When displayed like a rug in a gallery space, visitors are confronted with the choice of walking over or around the piece. This is evocative of literally walking over other people. Mounted on a wall the figures seem detached, almost mimicking colonial trophies on display. Both these aspects carry their own political meanings and critiques. Multilayered, complex connections can be made visible about experiences of movers and witnesses by using arts-based research. Artworks speak their own language and communicate what cannot be accurately disclosed in writing. They are open. They have another presence and life altogether.

From witnessing to moving and making with objects

By making public art using video film, painting and sculpting, I allowed my own witnessing and movement experiences to gain a public, visual appearance in their own right. My works aim to go beyond the parameters of the pedagogical or therapeutic situation into another realm: the public gallery, the exhibition venue and the private sphere of peoples' homes. The cycle from movement to making and traversing the private and public realms seems to me to generate different kinds of exchanges that can fertilise each other. By making films, paintings and objects, a personal response is invited from a public collective whose multiple eyes and minds I cannot know. Their perceptions, resting upon the surfaces of my canvasses and sculptures, do not register the motivations or associations that were my guiding principles. Instead, they make up their own selective readings and meanings. I trust that my objects speak independently of my embodiment for and through their own language of phenomena: through colour, texture, form and shape, art speaks for itself. The absence of my moving body from these objects dedicates freedom to those who view it, a liberty that is rarely experienced in performance where the audience always becomes party to what is on show. This independence of the visual artwork emerges in the transition between making and public display. Once on show, an object carries the intimate traces of the artist's moving and touching body into the public realm. It thus subtly yet publicly articulates the dance of making processes through its own objective manifestation.

When engaging in the act of painting on canvas my marks on the surface mirror my own movements. The depiction of another mover, whose features may come forward or retreat through me touching the surface with crayons, brushes and paint, transpires through the application of my own body in movement and interaction with the materiality of tools and surfaces. The painting itself becomes like an opaque mirror of my vision and movement:

myself and not myself, another thing and another body disappear and emerge. By using visual art I still obtain understanding and empathy for the body in its multifarious movements, gestures and facial expressions, but via a circuitous route. Instead of performing or choreographing my own or others' bodies, I communicate with the public via the traces of my movements now embedded within the visual records of film, painting and tangible objects.

One unexpected insight of my art-making process is the aforementioned interconnectivity between movement per se and movement in relation to the making and manipulation of an art object. Haptic experiences occur and are documented within visual arts and design, and I found that there are parallels to dancing as well. Coming from a dance and performance background I appreciate the fleeting visuality of moments of live movement. In the past I had thought of visual art primarily in terms of finished products and objects. Whilst movement and dance are of the moment, art objects often stay and retain their shape for much longer periods of time and hence have a completely different, repetitive effect upon the onlooker. Artifacts change over an altogether different time frame, such as a patina that gathers on a sculpture or a slow deterioration of materials such as wax or paper, and these processes can be part of the intended longer-term effect.

Initially in my arts-led research I had not considered how much the body of a maker is embedded in artworks alongside the textures and qualities of certain material characteristics. I learnt that movement enters directly into the making of visualisations, bringing up a whole new set of questions. How do the acts of movement themselves bear upon and determine the visuality of an art image? How do I choose and handle objects and materials? How does this handling bring me in touch with issues of a much larger ecological scale? How can turning my dancing attention and conscious embodiment to observation and working with objects inform and affect others?

Capturing the fleeting moments of seeing movement reveals a parallel reality of visual manifestations, influenced by the making with and through the body. For example, when using the particular physicality imposed upon me when holding a digital camera, I found myself to be both a witness and a mover revealing the relevance of embodiment and its effect upon and received from technology and its objects. I realized that using the 'third eye' of the lens within an apparatus does not alter the fact that it is me who directs and looks, a fact that is often overlooked when dealing with the astounding capabilities of cameras and other devices of visuality, such as drones. Influenced by the positioning of my body, choosing the perspective and at times moving with the other dancer, my images bear witness not only to her dancing but also to what and how I choose to see.

Experimenting with different tools and materials, from film to paint on canvas to making sculptures, designs and installations, I continue to note the various movement qualities known to me from dancing and the particular emergent relationships between their interactions with various materials. My moving, imagining body is the same in dance as in my movement interactions with the objects I craft, my moving is simply moving with materials. Haptic, sensory and kinaesthetic experiences of myself as a moving maker manifest within the made objects. Movement fixed into form reveals a poignancy of the mover's body in relationship to something else. The effect that the moving maker has on the material world is (another) testimony of the powerful influence that each one of us has through the gestural potential inherent in our bodies. We shape not only ourselves in movement but also what surrounds us, a well-known experience of improvisers in many different movement and dance forms, including Authentic Movement. But also social interactions of all kinds between moving bodies bear witness to the same principles. These influences are notable in the world of things and materials, within the design of daily objects and within the built environment, exemplified in interior design and architecture.

More images and details of arts projects can be accessed via www.share dhabitat.net.

References

Adler, J. (2002). *Offering from the conscious body: the Discipline of Authentic Movement.* Inner Traditions, Rochester, Vermont.

Arendt, H. (1958). *The human condition.* University of Chicago Press, London.

Atterton, P. & Calarco, M. (eds.) (2004). *Animal philosophy.* Continuum, London, New York.

Berrol, C. (2000). The spectrum of research options in dance/movement therapy, *American Journal of Dance Therapy*, Volume 22, No. 1, (pp. 29–46).

Deleuze, G. & Guattari, F. (2004). Becoming-animal. Atterton, P. & Calarco, M. (eds.) *Animal Philosophy.* Continuum, London, New York. (pp. 85–100).

Ehrenberg, S. & Wood. K. (2011). Kinaesthetic empathy: concepts and contexts. *Dance Research Journal*, Volume 43, No. 2, (pp. 113–118).

Foster, S. L. (2011). *Choreographing empathy, kinesthesia in performance.* Routledge, London.

Goldhahn, E. (2007). Shared habitats, the MoverWitness paradigm [Doctoral dissertation, Dartington College of Arts and University of Plymouth].

Goldhahn, E. (2009b). Visualising mover and witness: arts-based research. *e-motion, Association for Dance Movement Psychotherapy* (ADMP) U.K. 2009, Volume XIX, No. 3, (pp. 9–15).

McNiff, S. (1998). *Art-based research.* Jessica Kingsley, London.

Sperry, S. & Tsetse, L. (2003). Self and other, the practice of community long circle. *A Moving Journal*, Volume 10, No.1, Spring, 2003, (pp. 3–9).

Tsetse, L. (2007). Moving the outer rim in: Authentic Movement and non-violence. In Pallaro, P. (ed.) (2007). *Authentic Movement, moving the body: moving the self, being moved, a collection of essays*, Volume 2, Jessica Kingsley, London, (pp. 406–413).

Chapter 5

Being seen digitally: a filmic visualisation of a long circle in Authentic Movement

Introduction

Some of the ideas expressed in this essay were first published as a chapter in *Tanz & Wahnsinn - Dance & ChoreoMania* in 2011. Choreomania is a term describing an irresistible urge to dance and move and Birringer and Fenger's volume contains more than twenty contributions from dance research on the many ways in which dance can trigger an altered state of consciousness and, vice versa, how an altered state of mind can trigger dance movement. Choreomania provides an interesting, if provocative, term to look at the dynamics of a collective long circle in Authentic Movement. It poses that an interrelationship between consciousness and movement occurs in many different cultural contexts, historical times and geographies and how this phenomenon has met many different interpretations. In terms of Authentic Movement, choreomania is a moot and edgy term, something that might occur but is not intended by the practice. In this chapter, long circle, a specific practice format in the Discipline of Authentic Movement, is explored through digital *camera-witnessing* (Goldhahn 2007, 2011) in order to create a visual document that testifies an interdisciplinary approach using artistic and ethnographic research methods.

Choreomania

Choreomania is an uncontrollable urge to dance and move and some records of extraordinary instances of this phenomenon have been handed down from the early middle ages in Europe (Waller 2008a). Understood as possibly being caused by collective or individual experiences of disaster, dancing and movement spread from individuals to whole collectives and societies, taking hold of regions, towns and countries, whereby apparently hundreds were consumed by an irresistible urge to dance, hop and leap into the air (Waller 2008b). Choreomania, as described in Birringer's and Fenger's edited volume of essays, ranges from medieval villagers' uncontrollable dance journeys across the countryside to contemporary, urban flash mobs (Rohmann 2011; Stoye

DOI: 10.4324/9781003222309-7

2011). It can, apparently, take the form of Charcot's hysteric dance (Furse 2011) or be a dance of hysteria (Pape 2011). It occurs in the sophisticated forms of a Salentoean Tarantato (Manco 2011), in the whirling circularity of ecstasy and trance of mystical dances of the Sufis, and in idiosyncratic dancing of personal transformations in dance therapy (Weber 2011; Junge 2011). Contemporary choreomania can be witnessed at raves where, often under the influence of drugs, a mass of people dance ecstatically.

It may be argued that during her eight hour long performances the artist Marina Abramovic purposefully entered into a state of choreomania induced by her dance movement:

> I wrap my head in a black scarf.
> Performance.
> I move to the rhythm of the black African drummer.
> I move until I am completely exhausted.
> I fall.
>
> (Abramovic 1975)

Authentic Movement proponent Janet Adler in turn describes "mystical experiences" (Adler 1995) in connection with movement.

> I begin slowly turning in front of the fire, taking off my clothes. I scrape off, fling out, throw down, shaking my hands until they are numb, all the time turning, turning. Aggressive, loud sounds fill the room. My foot-work is precise, I spin faster and faster, creating a great circle around me, a circle of giant dolphin scales, clearest in the southwest corner. It is clear, all clear, between the edge and me.
>
> (Adler 1995, p. 111)

Joan Chodorow's presentation Movimento Authentico e Sviluppo Evolutivo Primario, at an event organised by "Art Terapia Italiano at University of Bologna (Chodorow 2003), elucidated a developmental approach to Authentic Movement". Explaining the interactions between movement and depth psychology, Chodorow also related some shortcomings that can occur in infant care. She then presented an Authentic Movement group session to promote embodied, experiential insights on this topic, with herself as the group's guide and witness. When some of the movement took on a collective dynamic, this session became one of the most powerful that I personally have encountered in Authentic Movement. Touched by the topic and feeling safe in Chodorow's presence, I gave myself permission to surrender to the proximity of other bodies, their rhythmic movements and their powerful soundings. Becoming part of a collective body that was warm, pulsating, sweaty, breathy and loud, I lost track of time. My inner witness still aware, I remember that I too made sounds, that I stamped rhythmically, that I was surrounded and held by other moving bodies and sounding voices. It now seems to me, that in the context of this circle of movers, momentarily, a form of choreomania manifested.

Authentic Movement's collective body

Authentic Movement encourages a conscious engagement with a semi-consciousness and allows movements to be spontaneous and 'authentic'. The movements arise from a state of day-dreaming (Payne 2003) and do not accord to any socially acceptable form of dance. Long circles can be the most commonly experienced practice format in Authentic Movement. Compared to other practice formats there are few detailed descriptive accounts of the workings of a long circle. Even Adler, when dealing with the subject of collective body, of which long circle is part, she does so more briefly than with other aspects of The Discipline of Authentic Movement (Adler 2002).

Yet long circle, and other collective body formats, have the capacity to enable experiences of spirituality (Adler 1999), evoke psychic contagion (Castle 2007) and even trigger psychosis (Elliott 2021).

> Certain words [like spirit] catch us in a contagious fascination. Such a psychic contagion is part of the mystery of the collective unconscious, as well as an outcome of media and technology.
>
> (Castle 2007, p. 275)

> I experienced two people on two separate occasions go into an acute psychotic break during an Authentic Movement workshop. This was not a class, it was an introductory workshop.
>
> (Elliott 2021)

Long Circle

At Somatics Festival (2019), Adler stated with regard to long circle that the only thing that is not allowed is to hurt yourself or another (Adler 2019). This is a central parameter and there are other aspects that contribute to making long circles safe. Long circles accommodate small to large groups of participants within one movement and witnessing session. A spacious circle, depending in size on the number of participants, is first mapped out by standing, and walking around it, in a ritualistic, meditative way. In long circle, all participants are either witnesses or movers depending on their own choice at a given moment. Alternatively, participants make an a priori commitment to enact only one or the other role throughout a session. Externally, witnesses can be identified by their position at the edge of the circle and their perceptive attitude of attention, their alert and watchful eyes. Witnesses remain either standing or seated, creating the space within which the movers perform. They consciously decide to observe the movers within the circle. Unless previously committed to remain a witness, a witness may become a mover responding to their inner impulse at any given time. A long circle can last up to 45 or 60 minutes. In theory, a mover can be a mover for the whole of a session or return to her place in the circle of witnesses at any time when she feels that a particular movement phase has ended for her.

As movers listen inwardly with their eyes closed, they are also responsive to a kinaesthetic and sonic landscape that is constantly changing and unfolding according to other individuals' inputs. Long circles "concern the deeper experience of membership in a non-hierarchical collective body" (Stromsted 2007). It is this interweaving of equal individual expressions into a whole group movement that is named the collective body, Adler's concept behind long circle.

The previously agreed ground rules of a long circle determine how many witnesses observe the group's movement at any time. This is to physically and psychologically safeguard the often deep and complex processes that can occur in this particular format. Yet the inbuilt uncertainty of who fellow movers and witnesses are at any given moment in time can add a powerful psychological element of not-knowing, one that requires a high degree of trust within the group and within each individual. Liminal psychological and emotional states, for example, dormant traumas, can give rise to heightened awareness and expressive imagination that an unprepared outsider could possibly perceive as choreomania.

Self-regulation

The group's process in a long circle usually regulates itself through each individual being able to choose her participatory role. A witness becoming a mover may substantially alter the direction and dynamic of a long circle. Movers can become moving witnesses, assisting and supporting each other and helping to regulate the emotional temperature of a particular long circle. The multiplicity of permutations of interactions between movers is seemingly endless. Inexplicably, groups tend to adjust to the psychological capabilities of those who are present. They are guarded by each participant's individual inner witness. Careful observance of safety rules, including the conscientious preparation and vetting of movers and witnesses, should be maintained. The potentiality of liminal states that a collective can enter together make long circle a very powerful practice, one that is open to new and unexpected experiences. It is the unexpected produced by the multiplicity of possibilities of a group and collective that can site a long circle within the realm of choreomania. In this realm, interrelationships are discovered as permeating and profound. Here, qualities of group-presence and embodiment, and a shared habitat of becoming a collective body, are a real possibility (Goldhahn 2007, p. 28).

Why film Authentic Movement?

Authentic Movement's long circles are usually protected in their privacy by mutual confidentiality. How can students or an interested public learn about or visualise a long circle? How can this format be researched? The film *Long Circle* aims to open an artistic and ethnographic window into this world.

My colleague dance therapist Marcia Plevin asked me to co-teach and make some film recordings of her Authentic Movement group in Finland some years ago. Co-leading Plevin's group facilitated my immersion in an unusual three-fold role as artist-researcher-teacher, similar to that of an ethnographer. The group's confidence in practising Authentic Movement was well established. The group's participants themselves had experimented with recording Authentic Movement using handheld cameras the previous year. I was welcomed with warmth and curiosity by the group and received their full consent and cooperation. Part of my process was to facilitate discussions, addressing participants' questions and concerns regarding my presence and the influence of the camera work on their personal practice. We agreed that group viewings of all the video rushes would be the prerogative to give permissions for publication. Hence all filmed material was vetted by participants. Could my approach to visualising Authentic Movement digitally in film be ethical and respectful enough to show participants' powerful, private work publically?

Being seen digitally: camera-witnessing

My inspiration for creating camera-witnessing (Goldhahn 2007) for filming Authentic Movement came both from the practice itself and from James Benning's very slowly moving landscape films shot from a single perspective. Camera-witnessing mediates the practice of witnessing: the perspective is still and altered only minimally, the camera, sited on a tripod, may move slowly or very occasionally focus in, emulating myself witnessing from a still position, turning my head occasionally to visually follow a mover in the circle. Not getting up and not moving around the space to achieve more interesting camera angles helps to provide the movers with the same sense of certainty as if I was a dedicated witness who is always known to be in the same place. Applying Wittgenstein's axiom that 'ethics and aesthetics are one' I adapted my filmmaking and my aesthetics to the ethics inherent in the Discipline of Authentic Movement. I simply became the witness with the camera. The resulting film is akin to an ethnographic or artistic document and gives privy into the usually sealed and private world.

In the film making of *Long Circle*, my perspective of filming was also determined by the difficult lighting conditions in the studio. Having windows at different angles, natural light had to be balanced with ambient interior lighting, resulting in graininess of the digital film. The editing process took place under the same premise as the filming itself, using respectful witnessing of movers' material. For the film I selected movement sequences that I felt drawn to. These were the memorable moments that a mover might have spoken about and that I might have offered verbal witnessing for. My editing from a 45-minute tape to an 11-minute film is, by digital filmmaking standards, an unusually small ratio.

In the studio of Authentic Movement practice, the camera and its lens can initially seem like a judging voyeur or a cold, surveilling digital eye. The authority given culturally to visual digital media, the camera, its lens and the one who yields this machinery, can seem to overpower, be considered depersonalised or even parasitic. The presence of a filming camera can feel as if something is taken away from the living moment itself. It is important to be mindful of such feelings and to make sure that the personal contact with participants, and not the dealings with the camera, are foregrounded.

Viewing the digital record, in turn, can evoke mixed feelings. When we reviewed the footage of *Long Circle,* most participants felt fascinated by seeing themselves as I had seen them via the camera. For some participants the footage provided additional confirmation of having been seen by me. Others felt that a filmic record was superfluous, as what mattered to them most was the lived, embodied experience and its memory. Some initially feared that something of their experience could be disturbed or taken away by seeing themselves and others on film, whilst others were curious to learn more. It was important to me that all participants' integrity was protected and honoured, and that when seeing the film each one of them should feel completely respected and seen.

The film *Long Circle*

The film *Long Circle* opens with one mover wandering and another mover performing a rhythmic and repetitive circular movement, propelling herself around her head with one leg pushing against the floor. Gliding around and around on the floor, the expression on her face is serene and happy. Another mover seems to be wandering with a sense of searching for a movement or standpoint. Soon, more movers join in, each one connecting to their own movement quest and displaying focus and concentration on their own activity.

Later, movers begin to connect in physical contact with each other and a new web of constellations and movements emerges. A configuration culminates in a figure of three movers ostensibly connecting and lining up

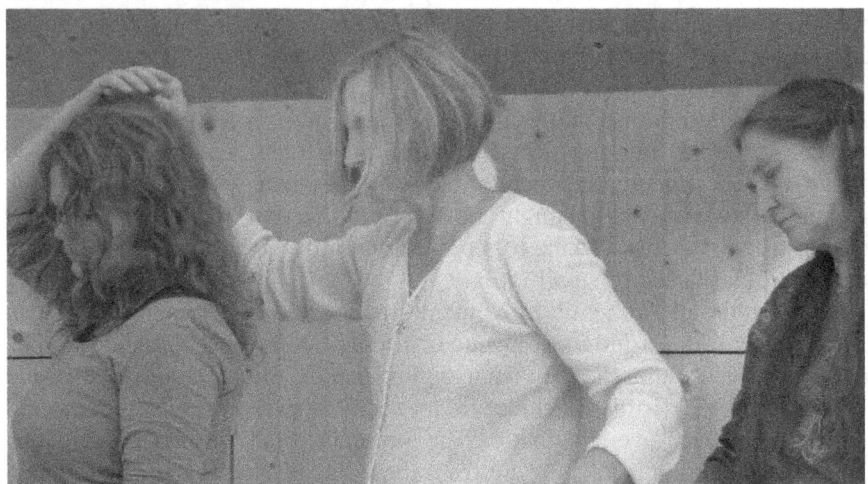

Figure 5.1 Three movers film still. Artist: Eila Goldhahn 2005.

in a tender and sensitive way. They stand with hands reaching and touching – forming a line with their heads tilted as if listening out for something. Indeed, at the same time, one of the other movers in the group has begun to sob deeply. Whilst from my personal witnessing viewpoint, the sobbing mover was not visible, the group's physical response and gathering towards this mover was.

Meanwhile, another individual mover was seen by me in a sitting position touching and moving her hands with concentration. At times, her face showed anguish that appeared to be linked to her pulling on her own fingers as if removing something that had stuck to them. With this activity intensifying, another witness entered the circle and reached with a caregiving gesture towards her. This was obviously unwanted, as I could now witness the seated mover moving away.

A little later, most of the group had gathered around, touching, holding and rocking a mover, that I cannot see from my position. At this point, I and the film look again at the handwringing mover. Gently lifting her head and opening the front of her body, she too seems aware of the distress of the unseen mover whilst remaining seated with her own hand movements.

Language and movement

I have used everyday phenomenological language to describe some scenes in the film *Long Circle*. However, languaging after the movement and transition time of a long circle in Authentic Movement has a well-set format in percept language, as explained in Chapter 3 of this book. It focusses on the use of verbs to describe actions to relate to oneself in the present tense and in the first person 'I'. Whilst this format of bearing verbal witnessing in Authentic Movement was developed by Adler (2002) it is preceded by Weir's percept language (1975).

In the 1960s, dance artists of the Judson Theatre, the birthplace of New Dance were already concerned with naming actions in a similar matter-of-fact manner. Also visual artists, such as Richard Serra, were interested in solipsism and the importance of doing as expressed in verbs. He created *Verb List Compilations: Actions to Relate to Oneself* (1967–68). Every observation, every feeling is theirs and no one else's. Preceding the practice of languaging in Authentic Movement both, this artist and this therapist, each in their own medium and way established a form of self-agency through language that is self-referential, not in a negative sense of being egocentric, but in a sense of being the agent of ones own perceptions of the world. Self-agency and a self-referential language can support an individual's mental health, aid their relationships and strengthen their self-image. In this way one is responsible for one's own perceptions and, in social conduct, does not project or blame these on another person. Languaging in Authentic Movement practices this by verbalising the moved and seen in a similar manner.

Interestingly, McCarren draws a parallel between dance and madness in that both seem to have their origin in an "absentia of speech" (McCarren 1998, p. 17). This can hold true when language and articulation of the self are completely suppressed and experiences may have no other way than to express themselves in movement. However Authentic Movement builds a bridge between the silence of movement and the languaging of movement in a complementary articulation of body and mind: a mover is seen moving and heard speaking. Language is inspired by and arises through embodiment.

When presenting the silent film *Long Circle*, I invite viewers to comment for themselves. The audience of the film is like a witness confronted with a vision of movement, having to find their own words and understanding of the seen. Authentic Movement can appear 'choreomanic', unusual, even strange to outsiders. *Long Circle* can provoke an initial state of speechlessness that leaves room for a search for words and comprehension. The omission of a speaking circle from the film does not condone an elimination of speaking from the practice itself but protects the movers' privacy. This lack of language in the film places the viewers into a meta-witnessing position. A situation is created in which experiencing the filmed, silent movement can precede an audience remembering, thinking and speaking about it. What is seen in the film could act as a basis to practice witnessing and languaging.

Viewers of *Long Circle* can use elements of percept language themselves such as sentences beginning with 'I see', 'I feel', 'I sense' or 'When I see this mover I can remember...' in order to describe their impressions, emulating a meta-experience of witnessing. Camera-witnessing, the method used to create *Long Circle,* has the potential to be used to create other digital documents. Films could be used in educational settings to teach Authentic Movement, especially when such teaching has to take place online. They should maintain the principles of safety and ethics in Authentic Movement practice (see also Chapter 11 of this book: Being seen digitally: micro and macro perspectives). Further, Marcia Plevin describes new developments in the Discipline of Authentic Movement

> Long circle, as practiced up until now, was considered to be no longer 'safe'. In the past, we tried to create a narrative in the speaking and witnessing of long circle and sometimes recognised that whole places and events were missing. Sometimes there were no or little witnesses present and the long circle simply generated too much unconscious material to hold and/or to process.
>
> (Plevin 2021)

I agree that silence can be a useful tool to honour forgotten events. By holding a silent space they still exist but remain on a level of the pre- or the post-verbal. Admitting and stating that 'I cannot name it' can be honest and respectful, whilst making a stronger demand on an individual's inner witness and their capacity to contain the seen, as in silent witnessing. Silence following movement can intensify prior movement experiences. Silence may contribute to the intensity of embodiment in movement (McCarren 1998) and, subsequently, can intensify its memory. Its different qualities seem to complement and contrast each other, and, according to Sheets-Johnson (2019), speaking from a philosophical perspective, a close interrelationship between movement and silence exists.

Choreomania pays tribute to dance's powerful, nonverbal origin that finds its ancient, embedded pathway through our nervous systems. To outsiders, Authentic Movement can temporarily give the impression of madness when this is absolutely not the case, as in the film *Long Circle.* Whilst I was not concerned about what does and what does not constitute so-called choreomania, the concept as an envelope for instances of seemingly spontaneous, 'authentic' movement is poignant, allowing a gathering of sources to place them into a dance anthropological context. When installed in a gallery, a film depicting movers and witnesses can be freely encountered by new meta-witnesses who can choose to see or not to see by staying or by walking away.

Conclusions

The term choreomania provides a thought provoking context in which Authentic Movement can be compared to and differentiated from dance expressions in which participants might completely surrender to unconscious forces. To safeguard participants' integrity collective body long circles take place within a vetted group, and are committed to develop inner witness capacity and a clearer understanding of oneself and others. Hence participation in a long circle evokes a set of individual and group responsibilities. Applying witnessing to film-making enables rare insights into this interesting work and might be used for training and arts purposes. *Long Circle* is a record of a particular session as seen from a personal witnessing perspective. Methodologically, this way of camera-witnessing aims to be congruent with the ethics of Authentic Movement itself. Documenting a perspective into a usually private world, *Long Circle* becomes an ethnographic, artistic document. Whilst such a document might express altered states of consciousness, it celebrates collective, embodied expressions in movement. It is Authentic Movement seen as an art form and films made in such a manner as *Long Circle* can share this understanding publically.

Acknowledgements

The credit for such intimate moments of movement goes to the participants of the group who permitted a rare insight into their dignified, personal performances. Thank you to the 'women of Pettu' and to Marcia Plevin for inviting this work.

References

Abramović, M. (1975). *Free the body.* In Abramović, M., Biesenbach, K. (ed.) The Artist is Present. Museum of Modern Art, New York, N.Y. (2010), (p. 88).

Adler, J. (1995). Arching backward, the mystical initiation of a contemporary woman. Inner Traditions, Rochester, Vermont.

Adler, J. (1996). The collective body. In Pallaro (Ed.) (1999). *Authentic Movement: Essays by Mary Starks Whitehouse, Janet Adler and Joan Chodorow.* Jessica Kingsley, London, (pp. 190–204).

Adler, J. (2002). *Offering from the conscious body, the Discipline of Authentic Movement.* Inner Traditions, Rochester, Vermont.

Anderson, M. J. (2005). James Benning's art of landscape: ontological, pedagogical, sacrilegious. Sense of Cinema *[online].* Available from: http://www.sensesofcinema.com/contents/05/36/james_benning.html. [last accessed 22 September 2021].

Birringer, J. & Fenger, J. (eds.) (2011). *Tanz und Wahnsinn, Dance & Choreomania,* Leipzig.

Castle, J. (2007) Calling Spirit home: how body becomes vessel for spiritual animation. In Pallaro, P. (ed.) (2007). *Authentic Movement, moving the body, moving the self, being moved. A collection of essays, Vol 2.* Jessica Kingsley, London, (pp. 274–282).

Elliott, W. (2021). Email to Eila Goldhahn, 7 March 2021.

Furse, A. (2011). Making a spectacle of herself: Charcot's Augustine and the hysteric dance. In Birringer, J. & Fenger, J. (eds.) (2011) *Tanz & Wahnsinn, Dance and ChoreoMania*, Leipzig.

Goldhahn, E. (2007). Shared habitats, the MoverWitness paradigm [Doctoral dissertation, Dartington College of Arts and University of Plymouth].

Goldhahn, E. (2009a). Is authentic a meaningful name for the practice of Authentic Movement? American Journal of Dance Therapy. Volume 31, Issue 1, (pp. 53–64).

Goldhahn, E. (2011). Being seen digitally: a filmic visualisation of a long circle. Birringer, J. & Fenger, J. (eds.) (2011). *Tanz und Wahnsinn, Dance & Choreomania*, Leipzig.

Goldhahn, E., Hämäläinen, S., Rouhiainen, L. (equal authors) (2010). Collective choreography: experimenting with a multi-modal approach. Embodiment of authority. Conference proceedings, Sibelius Academy, Helsinki.

Hämäläinen, S. (2007). The meaning of bodily knowledge in a creative dance-making process. In Rouhiainen, L. (ed.) Ways of Knowing in Dance and Art, Acta Scenica 19, Theatre Academy Helsinki. (pp. 56–78).

Junge, A. (2011). Tanzekstase und transformation. Die Eigendynamik des Tanzes als Transformation der Wirklichkeit. In Birringer, J. & Fenger, J. (eds.) (2011) *Tanz & Wahnsinn, Dance and ChoreoMania*, Leipzig. (pp. 151–165).

Manco, F. (2011). Bodied experiences of madness: a Tarantato's perception. Birringer, J. & Fenger, J. (eds.) (2011) *Tanz & Wahnsinn, Dance and ChoreoMania*, Leipzig. (pp. 264–283).

McCarren, F. M. (1998). *Dance pathologies: performance, poetics, medicine*. Stanford.

McNiff, S. (1998). *Art-based research*. Jessica Kingsley, London.

Olsen, A. J. (1993). Being seen, being moved: authentic movement and performance, *Contact Quarterly*, Winter/Spring, Volume 18, number 1. (pp. 46–53).

Pallaro, P. (ed.) (1999). *Authentic Movement: essays by Mary Starks-Whitehouse, Janet Adler and Joan Chodorow*. Jessica Kingsley, London and Philadelphia.

Pallaro, P. (ed.) (2007). *Authentic Movement, moving the body, moving the self, being moved. A collection of essays,* Vol 2. Jessica Kingsley, London.

Pape, S. (2011) Animal Magnetism – The dance of hysteria, the hysteria of dance. In Birringer, J. & Fenger, J. (eds.) (2011) *Tanz & Wahnsinn, Dance and ChoreoMania*, Leipzig.

Payne, H. (2003). Authentic Movement, groups and psychotherapy. *Self and Society – Forum for Contemporary Psychology*, Summer 2003, Volume 31, number 2, (pp. 32–36).

Plevin, M. (2021). Transcript of conversation with Eila Goldhahn, Email 15 May 2021.

Rohmann, G. (2011). Vom "Enthusiasmus" zur "Tanzwut": Die Rezeption der platonischen "Mania" in der mittelalterlichen Medizin. Birringer, J. & Fenger, J. (eds.) (2011) *Tanz & Wahnsinn, Dance and ChoreoMania*, Leipzig. (pp. 46–61).

Serra, R. (1967-68). *Verb List Compilations: Actions to Relate to Oneself*. Lepecki, (ed.) (2012) *Dance, documents of contemporary art*. Whitechapel Gallery, London, The MIT Press, Cambridge, Massachusetts.

Sheets-Johnstone, M. (2019). The silence of movement, a beginning empirical phenomenological exposition of the powers of a corporeal semiotics. *The American Journal of Semiotics*, Volume 35, 1–2 (2019), (pp. 33–54).

Somatics Festival (21 September 2019, video recording). *Panel 1, Why here, why then?* (Hosted by Olsen A. with Bainbridge Cohen, B., Adler J. and Starks Smith N.) Available online at https://vimeo.com/383359664 [last visited 1 March 2021].

Somatics Festival (21 September 2019, video recording). *Panel 2, Where are we now?* (Hosted by Adler J. with Bainbridge Cohen, B., Olsen A. and Starks Smith N.). Available online at https://vimeo.com/383373489 [last visited 1 March 2021].

Stoye, K. (2011). Die "Tanzwut"-Bewegung von 1374. Individueller Tanzwahn, tanzepidemischer "Flashmob" oder performativer Höhepunkt einer emanzipativen Laienfrömmigkeit? Birringer, J. & Fenger, J. (eds.) (2011) *Tanz & Wahnsinn, Dance and ChoreoMania*, Leipzig. (pp. 62–82).

Stromsted, Tina (2007). The discipline of authentic movement as mystical practice: evolving moments in Janet Adler's life and work, in Pallaro, P. (ed.) (2007) *Authentic Movement, moving the body, moving the self, being moved: a collection of essays*, Vol 2. Jessica Kingsley, London. (pp. 244–259).

Tetse, L. (2007). Moving the outer rim in: Authentic Movement and nonviolence. In Pallaro, P. (ed.) (2007). *Authentic Movement, moving the body: moving the self, being moved, a collection of essays*, Vol. 2, (pp. 406–413) Jessica Kingsley, London. (pp. 406–413).

Waller, J. (2008a). *A Time to Dance, A Time to Die: The Extraordinary Story of the Dancing Plague of 1518*. Icon Books, London.

Waller, J. (2008b). Falling down, *The Guardian* [Online]. Available from https://www.theguardian.com/science/2008/sep/18/psychology [Last accessed 20 May 2021].

Weber, A. (2011). Tanz als Therapie und Therapie für Tänzer: impulse aus Neurowissenschaft und Psychotherapieforschung. In Birringer, J. & Fenger, J. (eds.) (2011) *Tanz & Wahnsinn, Dance and ChoreoMania*, Leipzig. (pp. 131-150).

Weir, J. (1975). The personal growth laboratory: The Laboratory Method of Changing and Learning: Theory and Application. *Science and behaviour books*. K. Benne, L.P. Bradford, J.R. Gibb, R.D. Lippitt (eds.), Palo Alto, California. (pp.1–13).

Wittgenstein, L. (1984). *Tractatus logico-philosophicus*. Suhrkamp Taschenbuch Wissenschaft, Frankfurt.

Zuvela, D. (2004). Talking about seeing: a conversation with James Benning, *Sense of Cinema* [Online], available from: http://www.sensesofcinema.com/contents/04/33/james_benning.html [last accessed 22nd September 2021].

Chapter 6

Sculptural installations on the theme of obliteration: a response to themes embodied in Authentic Movement

Introduction

This chapter is based on an art essay first published in the *International Journal of the Arts in Interdisciplinary Practice* in 2009. It describes a project that visualised collective themes of death and loss, and is included in this book to show the process of transposition from qualities experienced in Authentic Movement into works of art.

Arts therapists (like arts teachers), whose primary focus is on helping other people to be creative, frequently neglect their own personal arts practices. Making art work for the public can seem outside of one's prime professional role. Yet it is one's own creativity and art-making that can benefit and sustain professional practice. Lack of opportunity or a sense of not being able to straddle both saddles of being an artist and an arts therapist (or teacher) can prevent such engagement. Creating public art requires a leap of faith.

In my enquiry into Authentic Movement, as part of my arts-led PhD (Goldhahn 2007), I explored methods and methodologies. How could I communicate aspects of my practice without compromising confidentialities? How could I express qualities of my witnessing in another arts medium? How could I write about these experiences? This artist's essay ventures into this realm of questions.

The choice of topic: obliteration

My sculptural installation *(Un)marked Boxes* transposes feelings of loss and images of death witnessed by myself in my primary practice, Authentic Movement, into public works of visual art. In 2005, three life-sized installations were created at Delamore Arts, Dartmoor and at Dartington Trust, Devon. Each one consisted of wooden crates arranged in different groupings and configured for specific locations. When reflecting and writing about the work, its background and its public reception, I use the term 'obliteration'. This is to express a deep collective fear of the destruction of human society.

DOI: 10.4324/9781003222309-8

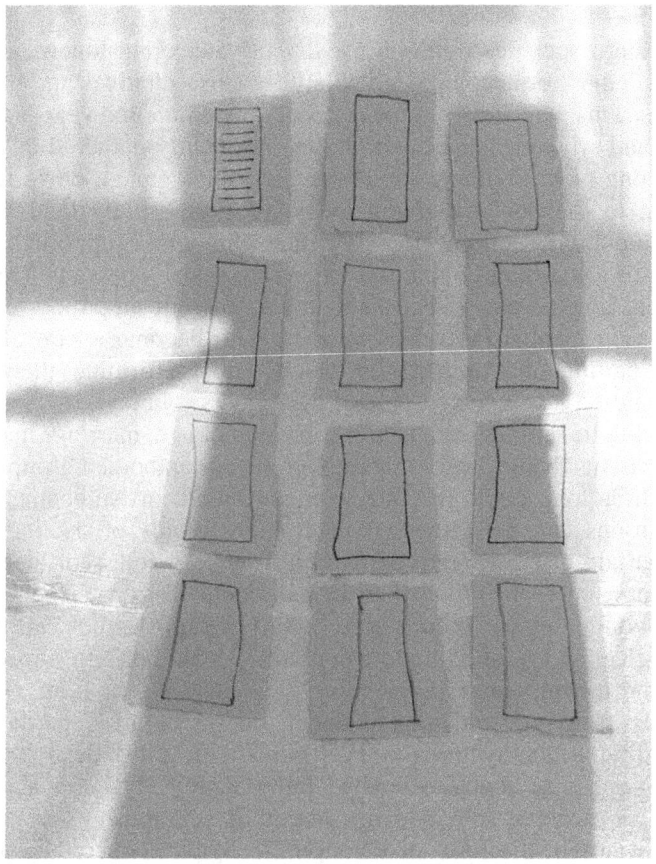

Figure 6.1 Sketch for *(Un)marked Boxes*, charcoal on paper on canvas.
            Artist: Eila Goldhahn, 2005

Topics such as individual death and collective obliteration are often shrouded from public view. In Western European societies these feelings tend to be held more privately than in other societies perhaps as a consequence of having closely experienced the traumas of two World Wars. Lately, in the face of accelerating climate change, pandemics and a new war in Europe, collective awareness of humanity's fragility has been painfully re-awakened and, as a consequence of these geopolitical events, has become more openly expressed. Prior to this, grief and fear of loss tended to be only shared in private family groups or in meditative or therapeutic groups, such as Authentic Movement circles. *(Un)marked Boxes* (2005) was created prior to these global developments, and was motivated by the wish for this topic of obliteration to be considered in a public sphere at that earlier time.

In Western societies dying is usually private; often lonely, avoided and unacknowledged or accompanied solely by close relatives and medical professionals. This was not always the case. A mere hundred years ago extended families and whole village communities frequently gathered at the time of death of one of their members. These gatherings gave a powerful sense of belonging to the person passing away, of being safely held within their own community. Coming together like this also supported the living members of a community at a time of an individual's passing. Thus communities were able to experience loss and a sense of emptiness consciously. Further, each member had the opportunity to become aware of their own eventual parting and prepare for death whilst affirming their aliveness. Death could be a less feared part of everyone's journey.

Major life transitions such as birth, coming of age, marriage and death frequently arise as themes within therapy groups or embodied group improvisations such as long circle in collective body work in Authentic Movement. Whole groups can be witnessed to embody rituals of decline, suffering, dying, burial, grieving and departure. I have witnessed these qualities emerge more often in group than in individual sessions. I believe that the sense of community of a collective body moving together can provide the psychological safety and support that individuals need to allow particular images and feelings to surface.

Broadly speaking death can be understood as the ultimate dissolution of individuality, a quality cherished as one of the most desirable values in secular Western societies. So-called individuality enhances a person with identity, professional role, socially important relationships, status symbols and even fame in the form of belongings, digital connectivity and wealth. Death then is a falling apart of what has been painstakingly built up during the lifetime of an individual and what has been largely relied upon. In death individuality has to be given up and surrendered. The individual body is the only carrier able to give organization to the values of the living. Each part, each limb, each organ, however perfect, beautiful, skilled, famous or loved, deteriorates, loses its perfection, its beauty, its skilfulness in order to become a mere ingredient in the potentiality of new gestation at another time and place. When being part of a group and with the mutual comfort and support available from others, it can be easier to give way to difficult and painful contemplations than on one's own. Authentic Movement's closed-eye practice can help to overcome inhibitions to collectively express grief together. It aids to maintain focus and a sense of individual privacy and dignity. Other societies more centred around a belief in the sacred often had more open, public ways to grieve and to prepare for death. I found that Authentic Movement circles and also art substitute the absence of collective public rituals.

Making *(Un)marked Boxes*

Authentic Movement circles can serve a particularly important function when providing space for difficult feelings that society has little space for. Art can serve the same purpose. I was in search of finding a way of transposing what I had seen and felt in Authentic Movement for public perception by using art. The creative process of turning these feelings and observations into art contained several stages: procurement, sketching, model making, trials and realisation.

(Un)marked Boxes were made possible when I obtained a large quantity of wooden crates from an industrial estate. The packing crates had been discarded and were crafted from new pine and unmarked except for a few stencils of arrows and the warning 'fragile'. Their shape, and size and pristine condition made them perfect ready-mades for my project. They would provide the building blocks for an installation with a modernist, stark, industrial aesthetic which I believed would provide an appropriate screen for a wide range of viewers' projections.

I experimented with one, two or three crates at a time, trying out different figurations such as leaning, stacking, and standing them upright. I moved around the crates to work out the shapes that I wanted to create. The upright crate became my favourite model as it reminded me most of the human figure.

Working two-dimenionally, I sketched their striking, oblong forms with charcoal on thick handmade paper, emulating the rough, sensory quality of the wood. Exploring these initial figurations evoked strong feelings within me. In particular, there was apprehension and anger. In my drawings the crates were empty. It was during this process that the stark association between empty boxes and death came to me. Confronting this association of death with emptiness was hard to bear. I titled the work after a line in a poem: "God's joy moves from unmarked box to unmarked box, from cell to cell" (Rumi, 1984, p. 46).

In the following phase of conception I made hand-sized models of the crates in cardboard and arranged these pieces on hardboard. Numbers of boxes and distances became important. How many, how far apart and in what configuration? Similarly, as when I had used paint on video stills exploring the notion of privacy and protection of a mover's image, I also began to veil the model boxes. Using gauze bandages as well as pencil and iron oxide red paint to draw, scratch and colour the surface on which they stood, again evoked strong emotions within me. War and obliteration became alive in my imagination and the act of drawing in particular became carthartic.

However, after working through that phase of exploration, I completely dismissed these additional elements of bandaging and colour as a visual language for my project in hand. I wanted to retain space, openness and a release for others to engage their own imaginations. I was not interested to display my own feeling process and I had no wish to use the public as a witness to my emotions and pain. Nor did I want to prescribe what others would think and feel, but instead I wanted to offer an open, if suggestive, space. Through the choice of the installations' prime elements, the crates, the topic of death was already suggested. Within the installations, I wanted to create a space that the public could engage with or simply walk away from. I also wanted to create an aesthetic that would not stifle or over-whelm, but that was neutral. Working out of doors and in the proximity of nature and its wholesome living shapes helped this agenda. From then on concentrating solely on the spatial formations, I narrowed my choices to three typical human movement groupings: circle, line and unstructured. I established spacings, proximities and distances between individual crates and thereby arrived at these three configurations. These were then shown at two different venues.

Delamore Arts, Dartmoor, Devon is a manor house with extensive grounds that hosts an annual sculpture exhibition primarily showing work by regional artists. Sculptural work is largely decorative and for sale. I introduced my, in this context unusual, concept to the owners and organisers and was offered a prominent space opposite the manor house for my installation. Here, again unusually, the owner had a Cromlech erected in 2000, a folly stone burial chamber ready for his own eventual burial. This monument in ancient style had been placed at the top of a lime tree avenue especially planted for this purpose, making a symmetrical and ceremonial design. I thought that this setting was perfect for my project, as it already contained a monumental piece, the cromlech, signifying its own purpose for death.

Half way along the avenue, I built *(Un)marked Boxes* in a large circle. In relationship to the cromlech, this configuration became associated with standing stones. Standing stone circles are still found locally on Dartmoor and in Cornwalll, and are compared to and actually used by circles of people coming together for ritual, observation of the skies and celebration of the change of seasons. These stone circles have the architecture of an open interior, a special place, a sacred space, a circle.

A large open space surrounded by upright elements infuses respect and a sense of the sacred. In addition to my circle of upright crates at Delamore Arts, I configured a couple of small unstructured groups between the avenue's surrounding trees. These could be seen before approaching and entering the main circle. A singular crate was placed on its own between the trees away from the main avenue partially hidden by low hanging tree branches. These figurations based on the individual figure suggested a coming to and going away from the large formal, circular shape. They suggested a dynamic between the individual and the collective, between informality and structure, and between the profane and the sacred.

At Dartington Trust, also in Devon, and also in grounds surrounding a very large house, Dartington Hall, I used different spaces for juxtaposing two formations: one of straight lines and another loosely structured in the form of a spiral. The Old Tennis Court at Dartington Trust provided a blank rectangular, open space, its history associated with the rules of the game and the movements of players. The court without its original markings was now empty and stark. It constituted a void: an empty moss covered flat tarmacked expanse. Curiously people avoided this space. They chose to circumnavigate it rather than cross it, even when this would have shortened their journeys to one of its surrounding buildings or to the garden beyond. Here in this space the crates for *(Un)marked Boxes* were placed on two intersecting lines at an angle of 90 degrees, creating the shape of a large arrow in the middle of the space. The crates were sited at irregular intervals, slightly softening the straight rigour of the overall design.

By the Gallery, a pleasant grassy and partially wooded slope next to the drive to Dartington's upper car park, is another unused public space. Its vegetation of small meditarranean pine trees and its topology suggested a place for the spiral shape albeit the slope presented a practial challenge. Here *(Un) marked Boxes* appeared to tumble down the slope whilst maintaining their humanoid uprightness. They made up a group of individual crates in friendly proximity to each other. When the installations were ready, sunlight and the resulting shadows created additional visual aspects. At The Old Tennis Court, the sun cast clear-cut, dramatic shadows on the tarmac doubling the material rows of crates. Low sunlight accentuated both the insides and outsides of the crates. At different times of day and in different weather patterns, visitors saw different visual impressions of the same works.

Moving: embodiment in making

The pragmatic realisation of *(Un)marked Boxes* required muscle strength, balance and spatial awareness. The only way I was able to move the boxes was simply with my body, they were too tall and unsteady to be trolleyed around. My method was this: I stood in front of the opening of a crate, gently tipped it over my curved back and, by straightening my knees and lowering my head, lifted its weight on to the arch of my torso. With my hands I steadied and maintained the balance of the crate. To set out the works I had to move each one several times until I chose the correct positions and uncurl to set the crate down. I had helpers too, so I could stand back to see the configuration and make adjustments. In order to steady the crates safely on site, we drilled small holes into their bases and hammered iron rods into the earth that anchored them in place.

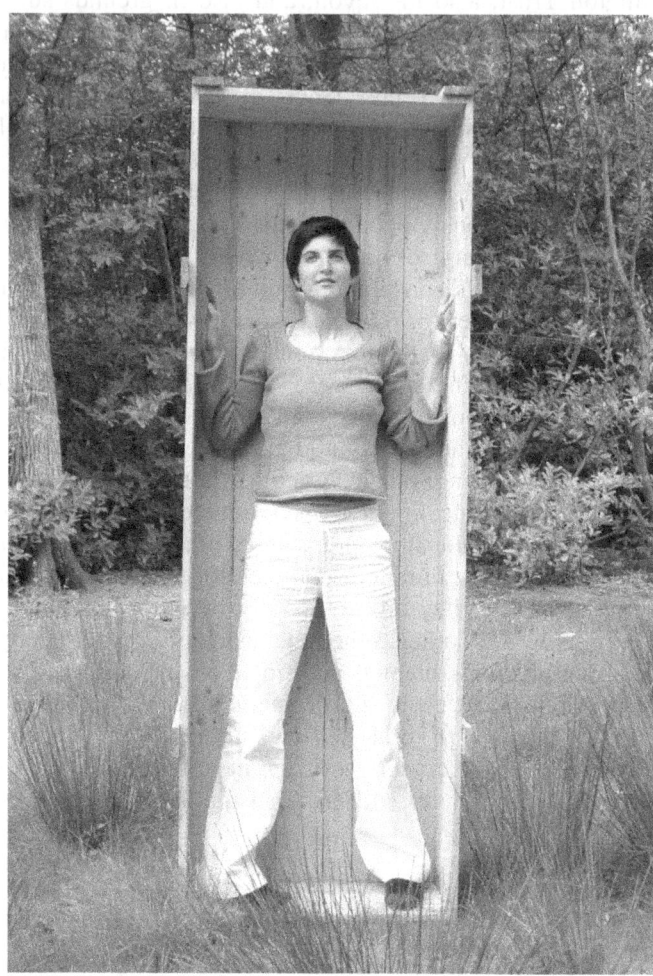

Figure 6.2 (Un)marked Boxes, site-specific installation with a dancer.
        Artists: Amber Burrow-Goldhahn and Eila Goldhahn, 2005.

Witnessing: conversations and interviews

On completion of these sculptural installations, my original witnessing of unplanned 'choreographies of obliteration' within Authentic Movement circles had migrated into a public sphere. Here the unexpected could once more take place, this time not by dedicated movers and witnesses, but by an audience. First I and my helpers, then other people entered and interacted with the circle and the other two configurations. *(Un)marked Boxes* provoked

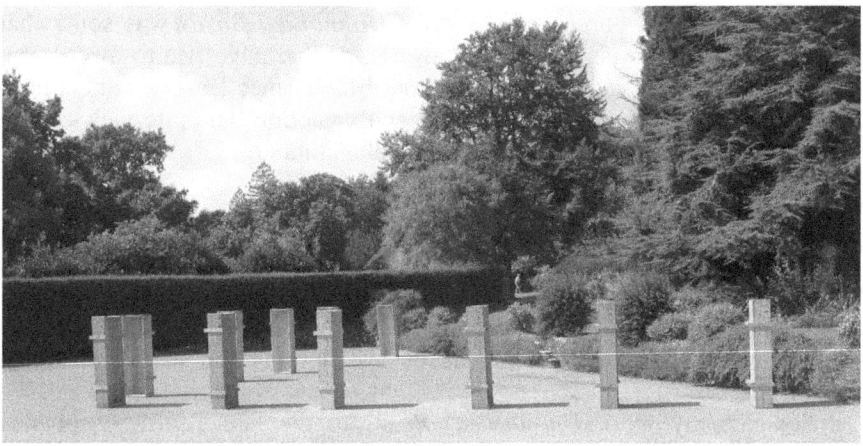

Figure 6.3 (Un)marked Boxes, site-specific installation: recycled, lifesize packing crates at the old tennis court, Dartington Trust. Artist: Eila Goldhahn, 2005.

and inspired strong and surprising responses, ranging from the thoughtful and amused to the shocked and touched. Whether playing hide and seek, or standing and dancing within a crate to feel what it is like to be within a wooden box, or simply feeling daunted to walk through the powerful circle of crates, visitors' experiences covered a wide range of feelings and associations. However I had not quite expected the public's vehement reactions when, one night, literal obliteration took place and youths pushed over a number of boxes, damaging their anchorage and altering the aesthetics of the designs.

Concluding thoughts

Private and public spaces come to life through shared experiences. The artist Joseph Beuys coined the term 'social sculpture' in the 1970s in order to expand on the existing notion of a sculpture to act as a socially transformative experience in the public sphere. Further, another parallel is in artistic process; "Beuys Actions [were] the starting point and source for many of his sculptures". (Rosenthal 2004, p. 100). Simply siting, constelling and public sharing transformed packing crates into becoming temporarily social sculptures. They were sites where individual and collective experience could come together. Once interacted with in the public realm, *(Un)marked Boxes* became works of art in their own right, independent of myself and my personal imaginations. They were performing a task mediated through their physical visuality and through people interacting with them. Making art is always accompanied by the experience of letting go, as the work quite suddenly belongs to the public sphere. Bringing the topic of collective fear of obliteration into the public sphere with *(Un)marked Boxes* was somewhat prescient as art often is. It raised an awareness that gave rise to discussion, interaction and even vandalism, a fact that I have since learnt can be a hallmark of a successful work of art! A film with reactions and interviews about this work can be accessed via www.sharedhabitat.net.

Acknowledgements

My helpers with *(Un)marked Boxes* were Stuart Young and Ben Burrow. Thank you Amber Burrow-Goldhahn, Anselm Ibing, Barbara Feldkeller-Weinstein and others for dancing in the installations and sharing thoughts and images.

I dedicate my work *Un(marked) Boxes* to the late Teresa Escobar. I remember Teresa with fondness in Adler's training retreats and again in peer group meetings.

Disclaimer

The author and artist affirms her right to her works *(Un)marked Boxes* described and depicted here and on her website www.sharedhabitat.net. These were made prior to a similar looking work by Antony Gormley as scenography for performances titled *Sutra*, which premiered on 27 May 2008 at Sadler's Wells, London.

References

Adler, J. (2002). *Offering from the conscious body, the Discipline of Authentic Movement.* Inner Traditions, Rochester, Vermont.

Goldhahn, E. (2007). *Shared habitats, the MoverWitness paradigm.* [Doctoral dissertation, Dartington College of Arts and of Plymouth, UK].

Rosenthal, M. with Rainbird, S. & Schmuckli, C. (2004). *Joseph Beuys: actions, vitrines & environments.* The Menil Collection, Houston with Tate Publishing, London.

Rumi, J. (1984). *Open secret.* Threshold Books, Putney, Vermont.

Part III

What is authentic?

Part III

What is authentic?

Chapter 7

Is authentic a meaningful name for the practice of Authentic Movement?

This chapter was first published in the *American Journal of Dance Therapy* in 2009 and is presented here with some edits.

Introduction

The term Authentic Movement is used in the fields of dance and dance therapy for a contemplative practice of movement, which for the layperson is primarily characterised by movement work with closed eyes and its observation by a so-called witness. Background to this work is Jung's concept of active imagination (Chodorow 1997), Mary Starks Whitehouse's , Chodorow's and Janet Adler's essays on Authentic Movement (Pallaro 1999). Further Adler's (2002) mystical approach formed the "Discipline of Authentic Movement", which gives specific directions for the semantic reflections and ritualised encounters between a mover and a witness. In the second and third generation of Authentic Movement teachers, many new variations of the practice have emerged and the term is often used non-specifically, meaning a host of loosely similar practices. In my writing, I refer to the work of Starks Whitehouse, Chodorow and specifically Adler, whose development I experienced during the 1990s.

Shared habitat

Like some other practitioners in the field, I believe that Authentic Movement is a movement practice of interaction and relationship that can build a strong sense of belonging and equality between participants. Whilst framing an equal playing field for all members of a group (witnesses and movers) the practice strengthens an individual's sense of identity. Authentic Movement demonstrates an exemplary view of a democratic exchange where each contribution, however unique, is valued by others. In Authentic Movement, each individual is accepted for his or her contribution to the whole, a notion exemplified in Adler's (1996, 2002) work on the collective body. To consistently value and respect individual uniqueness within collective experiences is a

DOI: 10.4324/9781003222309-10

rare and ethical element that has convinced me that Authentic Movement can have potential uses beyond the boundaries of movement and dance in other disciplines as well.

Instigated by my long-term experiences, especially with the collective body and by my interest in natural sciences, I have, in terms of my own practice and research, adopted a systemic perspective. In a biological and physical sense, the micro-level of cellular life and particle existence, and thereby of the human body, is influenced by and is part of what surrounds it. Viewed from this systemic perspective, the body has semi-permeable boundaries and exchanges take place with the environment (habitat) on multiple visible and invisible levels.

This perspective becomes especially apparent during group work in Authentic Movement, when movers and witnesses verbally exchange their perceptions, their shared habitat. By shared habitat I mean those moments in which movement and witnessing experiences meet (Goldhahn 2007). The careful linguistic separation and clarification of meta-levels of individual experience frequently reveal, enhance and unsettle interdependencies as well as respect for differences between participants. The revelations of varied realities conclude with a shared commonality between all participants.

The new insights thus derived weave a complex web of individual perspectives. Original viewpoints are not just seen as static and accepted, they are immersed into differentiated collectivity: they are necessary for the whole to appear. Akin to contemporaneous concepts in biology and philosophy, influenced by Deleuze and Guattari (1987), I think of all participants' experiences as being inspired and permeated, nourished and contaminated by a multitude of influences, a fact that can become apparent within and through the practice of Authentic Movement itself.

The unusual and expressive constellations in movement and word, which are frequently astounding and seemingly inexplicable in Authentic Movement, find in Levin's term of a "primordial choreography" possibly a fitting description. He states:

> For what we need is a thinking which actually deepens our contact with the choreography of the motility-field as a whole: a thinking which can actually take us into the depths of our topological attunement and help us articulate our felt-sense (our implicit, pre-ontological understanding) of the claim laid down for us in this primordial attunement. What we need, to put my argument in words is a thinking which can help us to reclaim our felt sense of being-open-to-Being as a way of being open, in our motility, to the grace of the field through whose clearing we move and pass.
> (Levin 1985, p. 104)

Can Authentic Movement provide a practical ontology to this quest? The questions of being, embodied through Authentic Movement practice, produce a choreography of the moment which evolves from unconscious to conscious. The unconscious, in juxtaposition and in connection with the term choreography, namely a consciously initiated form and composition, mirrors a difficult-to-grapple complexity.

Despite all this sharing of different habitats and immersions, clear boundaries and rules are typical and very important for the informed and successful practice of Authentic Movement. They lend form as well as psychological and physical safety. Yet also these spatial, temporal and psychological boundaries contain variables, ranging from movers' and witnesses' prowess, respective physical and psychological dispositions, to the time of day, the architecture of the space and the presence of other participants. Movers' and witnesses' perceptions and reflections are hence not solely attributable to a source within them but are made up of and modulated by the multiple factors that shape the topographies of their experiences. As in all ecologies, there are too many influences to name; that is why I pose that participants in Authentic Movement move within shared and permeable habitats.

Expressed in other words, and in naming the inherent paradox that follows on from the above premise, we can say that individual and collective movement, as well as spoken words, generate new memories and new knowledge. Yet, whilst weaving individual and shared meanings, movers and witnesses create patterns of complexity that can never be entirely complete. Even in skilful movement recall, it is possible to name astoundingly many, but never all, experiences. Something is always left out, missing, ignored or simply unnoticed. Each participant's ability to name phenomena remains limited to a particular frame of reality. Bound by the limits of language, participants probably learn to know no other site better than that of their moving, living body. Gaining detailed insight into oneself and one's interactions with others, that is knowing these shared habitats, is a journey supported and nurtured by the practice of Authentic Movement. But movers and witnesses alike, whilst generally satisfied with and motivated by the insights obtained, must also learn to accept imperfection, incompleteness and disturbances. This acceptance of not knowing, of paradoxes and their integration, is a very important, if not essential, part of this practice.

Questions regarding authenticity

In view of the above, the term authenticity evokes initially surprise and fascination. Associated with a true, inner place (Kemal & Gaskell 1999), the term authenticity implies a complete kernel of purity and truth, where disturbances and inscriptions from the world of phenomena are called to a halt. Whilst I feel in many ways attracted to this idealistic notion of the body and of the practice discussed as a vessel for authenticity, this concept is not compatible with my biologically and systemically oriented beliefs in which paradox and system create different parameters. Can the body be a site where the true being exists in an unchangeable, authentic form? Can Authentic Movement practice create a vessel for authenticity? Is the vessel whole or permeable, or is it both?

Psychological boundaries and clear temporal-spatial parameters in dance therapy and Authentic Movement play a crucial part in the psychological and physical well-being and safety of their participants. These boundaries are maintained and guarded in order to support a necessary and healthy sense of an everyday functioning reality. They also enable a temporary visit to an extraordinary perception of the self and the world, commonly identified as the unconscious. But is what movers and witnesses encounter within these boundaries more authentic than what is encountered without, or is it just more visible? Is the notion of authenticity compatible with the actual experience of moving 'authentically'? And, how can the mutually influential exchanges between movers and witnesses be described as authentic, or as 'not authentic'?

Reflecting on the term from a dance research perspective, Artus (1996) comes to the conclusion that 'authentic' offers great difficulties for the description of movement. He states that, even if it seems desirable to bring the identity-forming aspects of movement and dance to a centre of attention, the choice of wording 'Authentic Movement' remains unfortunate. On the one side, authentic is a term that cannot be enhanced. More than authentic is not possible! On the other, the development of a human being towards his/her authenticity is ongoing. We have the possibility to realise our own personalities until our death.

> Mary [Starks Whitehouse] explained the experience of authentic movement as one of 'being moved and moving' at the same time. As this balance becomes manifest, one begins to lose the illusion that one is anything other than one's body. In so doing, what is affirmed is the body, not the knowledge of the body or not the self. The body is not a symbol.
>
> (Adler 1985, p. 3)

Altogether, the concepts of fluidity and permeability are no foreign concepts in the practices of Authentic Movement; they resonate with the views of Jung, Starks Whitehouse and Adler. According to Jung (1940), feelings, emotions and affects arise and express themselves through our bodies, a notion widely accepted in dance therapy. Starks Whitehouse (1963, 1979) thematised the simultaneity of experiences within the consciousness of movers. She clarifies the inner dichotomy, which dynamically plays within the individual. One feels oneself to be moved and moves in an inner dialogue between initiative and receptivity. Widely drawing on comparisons with nature (notably water), she expressed a notion that could not better describe fluidity and permeability and which goes beyond any static notion of authenticity (Starks Whitehouse, 1958). The same applies to Adler (2002), who, by affirming the being a body rather than having a body, brings an alternative notion into play. If I am my body, and therefore completely permeated by my own bodyliness, it follows that I cannot contain a special inner core of authenticity. The body does not need an additional filling of authenticity, because it is not empty. The body is therefore already authentic. This would be in accordance with the widely accepted notion that the body cannot lie. Also, Jung's statement, "The symbols of the self arise in the depths of the body" (Jung 1940, p. 173), conjures up an image of permeability and not of a fixed site for feelings, emotions and images. These qualities instead arise. Yet none of these authors question (in keeping with the epistemologies that they moved within) the word authentic per se.

In my quest for clarification of the term, I associated the biological, osmotic movement of liquids from cell to cell with an authentic movement, namely a movement based in the biochemical and physical reality of organisms. In a geographical sense, the movement of a river from source to sea, creating its own topography, seems to me to be authentic. Here these meanings are aligned with a sense of the unavoidable, the inherent, the force of something stronger than something else that has the power to permeate and cross through whilst being a part of it. In the practice of Authentic Movement, mover and witness gather within a conscious and unconscious field: a shifting reservoir of involuntary, voluntary, knowable and unknowable, cellular and muscular phenomena. Following a natural science concept of permeability, I, as a conscious and unconscious mover and/or witness, can never know and name the constantly changing parts that constitute what I call myself. Consequently, all occurring movements and thoughts are authentic ones, not just certain specific ones, perceived to be authentic solely by some movers and/or witnesses.

It follows that this work always contains an element of the unexpected. One can never fully contain nor expel all (un)desirable occurrences within the practice of Authentic Movement. Instead one practises an attitude of openness and inclusion, whereby an element of the unexpected is factored into its workings. The result of this is a permeable continuum of moving and witnessing in which no separation between the authentic and the not-so-authentic is made. The practice of Authentic Movement is one way of developing knowledge of and through the habitat one calls oneself. But, because this habitat of I is in a constant state of flux, it is difficult to attach a specific quality to it. One cannot develop one's body or one's body's movements to be better sites of authenticity. In a sense, if we choose to use this ambiguous term, in the biological sense, one is already authentic and all movements are authentic. Authenticity is not a quality that can be measured on any scale by mover or witness and should be discarded as a statement used in witnessing.

Authenticity in other disciplines

In the arts, in particular, referents of the word authentic are associated with notions of being true to an origin (Kemal & Gaskell 1999). The word suggests the heritage, root and tradition of a particular piece of music, musical style or instrumentation, for example. Musicology, historical dance research and other cultural studies, when pursuing authenticity in their respective fields, are concerned with understanding and/or translating the traditional and historic documents of their particular art forms (Kemal & Gaskell 1999). However, the pursuit of traditional or historical movement or dance is not what the practice of Authentic Movement is concerned with. Although it could be construed that Authentic Movement chases after an original source of movement, in my view, it is rather concerned with the here and now.

A field of study closely associated with the term authenticity is that of aesthetics, which can be traced back to Aristotle's Poetics (Kemal & Gaskell 1999). In philosophy, scholars of aesthetics question and attempt to define notions of beauty. Beauty is a slippery quality to define and has often been associated with transcendent and/or religious experiences unique to humankind. When taken up by the spiritual texts of Islam and Christianity, religious transcendence became equated with authenticity (Kemal & Gaskell 1999). Whilst the practice of Authentic Movement is not explicitly associated with any religion, the experience of beauty is familiar to and treasured by many practitioners. This experience enhances motivation during the at-times arduous tasks of witnessing and aids the development of understanding, clarity and empathy between movers and witnesses. Adler's pedagogy of the Discipline of Authentic Movement, in particular, braids the true, the beautiful and the spiritual into one. In addition, various practitioners' contributions to *A Moving Journal* (1996–2004) express sentiments demonstrating respect for transcendent encounters enabled by the practice of Authentic Movement.

In *The Body's Recollection of Being*, Levin (1985) poses that the body remains the one place where, despite traditions, inscriptions and scripts unauthored by ourselves, we may still feel like ourselves. With this, he too turns the idea of authenticity into something less than absolute. His writings resonate in many crucial ways with my understanding of the practice of Authentic Movement. For example, I share Levin's sentiment that the body's recollection, particularly of movement, helps to reinforce a sense of identity. However, Levin suggests that conscious embodiment is a journey that can lead towards a core goal, namely towards the 'authentic'. Although

Authentic Movement can be understood as a journey, it has no definitive or final goal. Its predominant quality is movement in the present time and, as such, is antithetical to the idea that another constant or ultimate aim or place of perfection exists. Instead, I suggest that the practices of Authentic Movement explore the rich and living presence of varied, permeable and fluctuating habitats.

From philosophy to commoditization

Different schools of thought have questioned and scrutinised the concept of authenticity. Members of the Frankfurter School (Horkheimer & Adorno 1947), for example, highlighted the fact that the authentic was exploited as an idealised and absolute notion under fascism in the first half of the 20th century. Both Adorno (1973) and Benjamin (Buck-Morss 1991) critically assessed the term authenticity and the notion of timeless truth. Instead of adopting the notion of authenticity to describe the true, truth is regarded as bound to history and societal influence.

The socio-cultural influences of a specific time and place also contextualise what is conceived of as truth within the practice of Authentic Movement. Not only are concepts, opinions and views expressed within the signs of language relative to perspective and interpretation, but so also is the direct experience of the body in movement. So whilst the body may still be a place where we feel to be ourselves, as stated by Levin (1985), this experience simultaneously underlies the permeating function of time and context.

As a result of the widespread uptake of the writings of the Frankfurter School, many artists and scholars share, at times, a critical perception of the notions of the authentic and the original. Yet whilst being intellectually passe´ these attributes have in recent years been rendered fashionable in our capitalistic contemporary cultures. It seems that marketing strategies exploit the widespread spiritual and philosophical voids felt within and have answered with a backlash of authentic products for sale.

People have long had a liking for the look, sound and taste of something that originates from a culture other than their own, from the Indian curry to the Scottish kilt. Whilst global market strategies have successively eroded regional diversity, high sales figures are now obtained on products that simply claim to be, and are called, authentic. As people feel compelled to buy an increasingly diminishing sense of uniqueness, the word has become a favourite attribute in product labelling (Authentic Clothing Company, Authentic Foods, Authentic Jeans, Authentic Breathing Exercises, Authentic Handbags, Authentic Pine Floors, Authentic Education, Authentic Business). Promoting a false sense of authenticity, i.e. one that is globally mass-produced, the quality itself, once associated with truth, beauty and spirituality, has been degraded and ridiculed. This is the result of a homogenising international economy in which purchasing power is mingled with the desire to be recognised, individually and collectively.

Conversely, the Discipline of Authentic Movement has (so far) refused commoditization. The attempt to trademark the term in Germany in 1998 failed its intention. After initially supporting the formation of a German training centre (which would have required that the term Authentic Movement be trademarked), Dr. Janet Adler, Dr. Joan Chodorow, Neala Haze, and Dr. Tina Stromsted (1997) did not like the idea to protect the name by law and subsequently resigned as its trustees. Other groups, (such as La Luna, an international peer group, and the Italian Authentic Movement practitioners contingent, and others) spoke against such a commoditization of the term. Trademarking is common in other somatic practices (for example Body Mind Centering®, Skinner Releasing Technique™ and others), yet interestingly in the Authentic Movement community, it was critically discussed and eventually rejected.

Whilst it could be said that dance therapy and the practice of Authentic Movement are purchasable practices sold by professionals, they can imbue participants with a real, embodied sense of uniqueness and belonging. Furthermore, and to my mind especially important, the practice of Authentic Movement is self-reflective and creative. It has the tools to examine and interrogate the very concepts of individuality and collectivity, an important task in confronting the confusing challenges of human commoditization.

As Chodorow (2005) mentioned to me personally, the practice of Authentic Movement teaches one to become and remain an individual within a collective. At a time when international market economies have reached what is possibly their final round of ruthless exploitation, potentially causing great upheaval and disturbance within human and non-human systems, this particular pedagogical merit of the practices of Authentic Movement can be of great relevance and help. Despite loud academic and artistic challenges, the authentic product is an ongoing sales hit. Whilst the experience of individuality may be eliminated through boundless, collective consumerism, the word authentic should be used with care and circumspection. Its use can lead to a series of difficult-to-dissolve misunderstandings or wrong expectations which are to be best avoided by those who practice Authentic Movement wisely.

Teaching Authentic Movement

Barthes (1967), with his seminal essay Death of the Author, poses that author and script should be considered as separate entities, with a search for meaning always being a disentanglement rather than a deciphering. I see the process of disentangling and naming the web of movements in Authentic Movement similarly as a function of the witnesses who, independently of movers' personal histories, do not seek for the origin or reason of movements, but for the associations engendered within themselves; they seem like readers of textures of movements. They do not interpret or decipher movement but instead trace what has been seen and try to grasp and hold the seen within words. They approach the text of the mover through their own embodiment and language. That, what emerges within the network of relationship, within the exchange between mover and witness, no longer belongs individually but emerges as a communicative interaction.

In my personal experiences of Authentic Movement, all forms and derivations of movement are acceptable. There is no authenticity yardstick to compare a desired quality with an unwanted quality of movement. In fact, there is no right or wrong movement. Rather, the practice sets up a non-judgmental framework, which focuses on the relationship between observer and observed, listener and speaker, mover and witness. This relationship is characterised by a welcoming acceptance of whom and what the other is and does. This acceptance I understand to be an integral part of the essence and intention of the practice: it enables different perceptions of the same movement event to exist side by side. Methodologically speaking, this is an important assumption and one that I am particularly interested in. It is an epistemological cornerstone, so to speak, a paradigm that bears consequences for how we think about what we do when we engage in the practice.

In many forms of psychotherapy the term authentic is part of the professional jargon when speaking about self and clients; whilst innocuously adopted, it can be a subtle way of passing judgement and assessment on another. Often the speaker is unaware of in fact attributing projections onto somebody else when supposedly an expert's opinion is being expressed. A statement such as 'you seem to be really authentic in this moment', although given with the best of intentions by expert or novice alike, is, at first sight, a positive even a supportive one, yet it is in my view misplaced. Such statements may not meet the experience of mover or witness, but more problematically, they pass implicit judgement and undermine the principles of Authentic Movement (or those of humanistically oriented psychotherapies). For example, 'I feel close to my own expectations and hopes when I see you' may be a clearer alternative.

As I discovered through investigating the varied meanings and conceptions of the word, calling something 'authentic' is a qualitative statement. Having wide-ranging associations, meanings, assumptions, and most importantly, carrying implicit value statements, it should thus only be adopted with utmost circumspection. If something is deemed 'authentic' we tend to trust and believe it without reflection. We value all things authentic as this term touches on notions of an innermost truth and its associated beauty, a potentially seductive mixture. The actual perception of authenticity, and that what moves us, is always a personal experience, inculpable of static judgement, which, if stated, would destroy an experience smitten to a singular moment in time. Therefore, it is the privilege and the duty of witnesses and pedagogues to utter such experiences sensitively and responsibly.

New students of Authentic Movement often, and quite understandably, ask me as a teacher and witness whether they move authentically; in response, I explain that this is not a useful question to play with as it may prevent a mover from engaging with the status quo of their movement exploration. Yet the practice's prevalent name naturally attracts the mover who wants to learn how to move (more) authentically. Yet, and seemingly in contradiction with its name, in Authentic Movement all movements are acceptable, correct and right as they appear! A witness's purposeful speech is nonjudgmental of the mover. However, authenticity becomes a currency and as such a weighty burden when used by students who wish and desire to get rid of or move beyond the inauthentic. The desire for acquisition of authentic movement is an expression of becoming better at it and is, in my own and other colleagues' views, a hindering rather than a supportive or liberating notion to engage with. I do not become myself, I already am myself and hence, I am authentic. This is what I impart to my students. The need 'to be seen' is close to the essence of this work and is often the reason why people are attracted to it. Unfortunately, here also the term authentic movement can be a hindrance rather than a blessing.

Whilst being not immune to the pleasures of beauty in my perceptions as a witness (I am also an artist!), as a pedagogue I do not find this or the notion of authenticity useful parameters to engage with. Perhaps, and in view of such dilemmas, the sobering definition of authentic as "cognisance of meaninglessness of the world, yet deliberately follow[ing] a consistent course of action" (Chambers 20th Century Dictionary 1983, pp. 81–82) is perhaps an outdated, but usefully provocative notion worth pondering.

The MoverWitness

Despite the critical reflections outlined above, the name Authentic Movement remains useful when identifying particular practices in their historical and cultural contexts. It enables others to identify the lineage of teachers and peers that have taught and passed on these practices. The Discipline of Authentic Movement clearly belongs to Adler's (2002) terminology and I am especially indebted to her teachings.

During my investigations into the terms 'authentic' and 'authenticity', I uncovered multiple subtle, interesting as well as misleading referents and interpretations, mostly incompatible with how I understand the practice to work. The rationale for renaming my own practice is hence based on my conception that the operative principles within Authentic Movement form a paradigm made up of equality, permeability and complexity. Whilst a specialised biological interpretation of the label authentic movement would fit my own readings, this little known meaning would be difficult to communicate within cultural and interdisciplinary studies at the present time. These findings have persuaded me to propose an alternative name: the MoverWitness.

The composition of this new name arose out of my own deconstruction and analysis of Authentic Movement practice. The reason for choosing to write the words mover and witness as one word (MoverWitness), without a space separating the two nouns, lies in my desire to show the interconnectivity that I perceive to be at the heart of the practice: without mover, no witness; without witness, no mover. Using the capital letters indicates their unwavering individuality within their shared habitat.

Whilst my new term may not entirely express in words the ingenious elegance of the actual embodied practice, it serves research trajectories and teaching purposes more accurately. Self-perceived and other-perceived realities can approach each other through the equal exchange between movers and witnesses.

References

A Moving Journal. (1996–2004). Retrieved from http://www.movingjournal.org/ [last visited 2015]

Adler, J. (1985). Who is the witness? A description of Authentic Movement. (pp i–23). Self-published copy. Dated November 1985.

Adler, J. (1996). The collective body. Pallaro, P. (Ed.). (1999). *Authentic Movement: essays by Mary Starks Whitehouse, Janet Adler and Joan Chodorow* (pp. 190–204). Jessica Kingsley, London.

Adler, J. (2002). *Offering from the conscious body, the Discipline of Authentic Movement*. Inner Traditions, Rochester, Vermont.

Adler, J. (2004/2005). E-mail correspondence with the author (excat date and year?).

Adler, J., Chodorow, J., Haze, N., & Stromsted, T. (1997). Open letter. *A Moving Journal*, Vol. 4, No. 3, (1997), (p. 9).

Adorno, T. (1973). *The jargon of authenticity*. Routledge & Kegan Paul, London.

Artus, H. G. (1996). Authentizität, Authentische Bewegung und Tanz. , H.-G., Berger, F. R., Rosenberg-Ahlhaus, C. & S. Trautmann-Voigt, S. (Eds.) (1996), *Jahrbuch Tanzforschung*, Heinrichshofen-Bücher, Wilhelmshaven, (pp. 176–194).

Barthes, R. (1967). The death of the author. *Aspen: The Minimalist Issue, 5/6*. Retrieved from http://www.ubu.com/aspen/aspen5and6/threeEssays.html#barthes

Buck-Morss, S. (1991). *The dialectics of seeing: Walter Benjamin and the Arcades Project*. MIT Press, Cambridge, MA.

Chodorow, J. (1997). *C.G. Jung, Jung on active imagination, key readings selected and introduced by Joan Chodorow*, Routledge, London.

Chodorow, J, (2005). Note to Eila Goldhahn, 14 October 2005.

Deleuze, G., & Guattari, F. (1987). *A thousand plateaus: capitalism and schizophrenia*. University of Minnesota Press, Minneapolis.

Goldhahn, E. (2003). Authentic Movement and science. *A Moving Journal.* Volume 10, No. 3, (pp. 12–15).

Goldhahn, E. (2007). *Shared habitats, the MoverWitness paradigm.* [Doctoral dissertation, Dartington College of Arts and University of Plymouth, UK].

Horkheimer, M. & Adorno, T. (1947). *Dialektik der Aufklärung, Philosophische Fragmente.* Querido, Amsterdam.

Jung, C. G. (1940). *The psychology of the child archetype. The Collected Works of C. G. Jung* (Vol. 9, Part 1, pp. 151–181) (1969). Princeton University Press, Princeton, NJ.

Kemal, S. & Gaskell, I. (1999). Performance and authenticity in the arts. In S. Kemal & I. Gaskell (Eds.) (1999) *Performance and Authenticity.* Cambridge University Press, Cambridge, (pp. 1–12).

Kirkpatrick, E. M. (1983). *Chambers 20th Century Dictionary.* Chambers Harrap Publishers, Edinburgh, UK.

Levin, D. M. (1985). *The body's recollection of being: phenomenological psychology and the destruction of nihilism.* Routledge & Kegan, London.

Pallaro, P. (ed.) (1999). *Authentic Movement: essays by Mary Starks-Whitehouse, Janet Adler and Joan Chodorow.* Jessica Kingsley, London and Philadelphia.

Starks Whitehouse, M. S. (1958). The Tao of the body. In Pallaro, P. (ed.). (1999). *Authentic Movement: essays by Mary Starks Whitehouse, Janet Adler and Joan Chodorow* (pp. 41–50). Jessica Kingsley, London.

Starks Whitehouse, M. S. (1963). Physical movement and personality. In Pallaro, P. (ed.). (1999). *Authentic Movement: Essays by Mary Starks Whitehouse, Janet Adler and Joan Chodorow* (pp. 51–57). Jessica Kingsley, London.

Starks Whitehouse, M. S. (1979). C. G. Jung and dance therapy: two major principles. In Pallaro, P. (Ed.). (1999). *Authentic Movement: Essays by Mary Starks Whitehouse, Janet Adler and Joan Chodorow* (pp. 73–101). Jessica Kingsley, London.

Chapter 8

Towards a new ontology and name for Authentic Movement

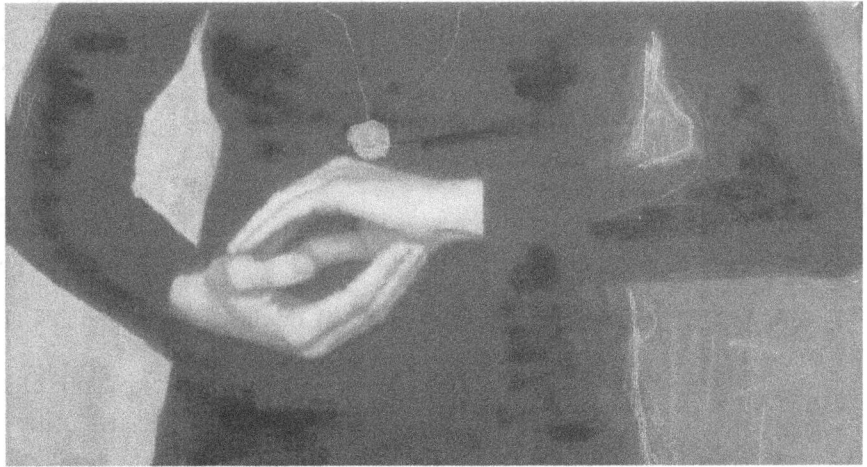

Figure 8.1 Holding hands, paint on film still. Artist: Eila Goldhahn, 2005

This chapter is based on an essay first published in the *Journal of Dance & Somatic Practices* in 2015.

Introduction

Authentic Movement is a practice of conscious embodiment that can be understood as being present with 'movement and stillness', and with 'being seen and seeing'. Mover and witness are the key players in this work. In the 1990s, American proponent Adler conducted annual retreats in the emerging Discipline of Authentic Movement in Italy and in Greece. During these retreats, an invited group of about twenty dancers, dance therapists, psychotherapists and somatic practitioners practiced under Adler's

DOI: 10.4324/9781003222309-11

guidance. Usually starting the retreats with work in dyads, consisting of one mover and one witness, and progressing to group work, where Adler and an assistant were the sole witnesses and all participants were movers, the retreats developed into formats such as breathing circle and long circle. When these retreats had come to an end in 2001, these formats were described in detail in Adler's primer *Offering from the Conscious Body, The Discipline of Authentic Movement* (2002). The author of this article participated in most of these retreats, and references Adler's very specific formats (see also Chapter 3).

Whilst being positively aligned to Adler's practice this article builds on the preceding Chapter 7 and takes a critical look at the practice's name 'authentic' and its underlying assumptions. It explores what may be taken for granted or even misunderstood. As Authentic Movement practice evolves through new generations of practitioners and students, it reflects on the relationship between assumed and actual meanings and their related philosophies. Thereby it questions underlying and presumed ontological certainties, entering into a reflective process that considers a contemporary, critical understanding

> Any accusation of betrayal necessarily implies the reification and reaffirmation of certainties in regard to what constitutes the rules of the game, the right path, the correct posture or the appropriate form of action. That is, any accusation of betrayal implies an ontological certainty.
>
> (Lepecki 2006, p. 1)

Starks Whitehouse's (1958, 1963, 1979), Chodorow's (1991) and Adler's (1987, 1996, 2002) texts are pointers to initial reflections on the term 'authentic' in relationship to movement. The term is then traced within dance and develops a critique making reference to the philosophical use of this term in Heidegger and Adorno. It then explores the problematic implications of the term's post-colonial and digitised meanings.

> As I discovered through investigating the varied meanings and conceptions of the word, calling something 'authentic' is a qualitative statement. Having wide-ranging associations, meanings, assumptions, and most importantly, carrying implicit value statements, it should thus only be adopted with utmost circumspection. If something is deemed 'authentic', we tend to trust and believe it without reflection. We value all things authentic as this term touches on notions of an innermost truth and its associated beauty – a potentially seductive mixture. The actual perception of authenticity, and that what moves us, is always a

personal experience, inculpable of static judgment, which, if stated, would destroy an experience smitten to a singular moment in time. Therefore, it is the privilege and the duty of witnesses and pedagogues to utter such experiences sensitively and responsibly.

(Goldhahn 2009a, p. 61)

The second half of this chapter identifies and explores some of the practice's key methodological qualities. These, it is posed, may serve as a basis towards a new ontologic understanding of the practice. Concluding, a renaming of Authentic Movement practice is, again, proposed (Goldhahn 2007, 2009a, 2010a). A case is made for a term that more closely reflects the actual methodological workings of the practice expressing the view that contemporary philosophies are well suited to support this.

The origins of the term authentic movement

The term 'authentic' can evoke confusing feelings and associations. It is popularly used in commercial contexts selling products and services that purport to be homey and special. A slippery term, proponents of Authentic Movement such as Adler and Chodorow, and myself, have felt discomfort that the term does not do justice to this rich and profound practice. In the Discipline of Authentic Movement, as in the MoverWitness, as in most other forms of Authentic Movement, all forms of movement and stillness are acceptable. Why do 'authentic' and 'movement' stand together in a name and purport to be the practice's prime characteristics?

Following this question historically, within the field of dance and dance therapy, it emerges that American critic John Martin appears to have first used the term 'authentic' in relationship to dance in 1933. Martin appears to have drawn the word 'movement' and the word 'authentic' together in one descriptive term. He related this combination of words to Mary Wigman's German expressionist dance performed in New York. Martin says "the first result of such creation is the appearance of certain entirely authentic movements" (Martin 1965, p. 59). Martin's application of the term authentic movement was in response to seeing Wigman's highly emotive, expressionist dance *Hexentanz*, one in which the dancer's soul appeared to expose itself through emotionally charged dance movements and gestures.

Starks Whitehouse's writings from the 1950s to 1970s, exemplify her own search for a language that describes what she found to be at the heart of the dance and movement that she enabled her students to find for themselves in her studio. Naming her studio practice 'movement in depth', Starks

Whitehouse was influenced by Jung's concept of active imagination combined with its embodied expression in movement and dance. This was developed by proponents Adler, Chodorow, Haze and Stromsted, who became the first generation of trainers of Authentic Movement in the USA (1996). Starks Whitehouse's work slightly preceded American post-modern dance (Banes 1980 & 1993) and there is a parallel between the inward-looking, self-directed nature of then newly evolving approaches to dance improvisation such as Release Dance.

Wigman, Starks Whitehouse and her students Adler and Chodorow; and American post-modern dancers such as O'Donnell Fulkerson and Paxton, all developed a strong awareness of creativity and the power of the imagination and looked for ways to access and manifest this in their respective dance forms.

German expressionistic dance garners images for their emotional power resulting in dance works that are raw and intense and bringing normally unconscious content to the surface of performance. Using repetition, amplification and testing the limits of capabilities of body and mind, it produced what Martin called 'authentic' movement.

Starks Whitehouse and her students originally also used repetition, amplification as well as stillness, an awareness of the body and mind. It seems that the integration of these elements was used to elicit movement that seemed authentic and therefore was at times perhaps alike to Wigman's dancing. The difference was, that Starks Whitehouse work was not produced for the purpose of public performance but to develop movers' ability to be themselves in movement and in stillness. Conversely, post-modern dance used sensation and stillness as a starting point for imaginative dance improvisation (O'Donnell Fulkerson 1982). Performance did not focus on or amplify emotions. (Paxton 1981a).

Whatever the differences in some of these historically close dance developments were, it appears that Adler actually coined the name Authentic Movement for the practice first in her essay Who is the Witness first circulated privately from November 1985 and then published by *Contact Quarterly* in 1987. Following subsequent years of practice and development, her primer of 2002 names the practice as The Discipline of Authentic Movement. Adler muses that perhaps a connection was woven in 1933 between Wigman's dancing in New York, Martin's attending and critiquing these performances and her own teacher Starks Whitehouse's developing practice. Adler wonders that Starks Whitehouse might well have been familiar with Martin's work and might have picked up on the combination of these terms (Adler 2002). However, Martin's notion of the 'authentic' was possibly equally informed by Konstantin Stanislavski's method for actors and the increasingly influential persuasively beautiful philosophy of German philosopher Martin Heidegger.

The philosophical term authentic

Heidegger was Edmund Husserl's student, who was the founder of phenomenology. Heidegger became Germany's most prominent philosopher in the 20th century. Phenomenology is a branch of philosophy that examines the development and the use of language. Heidegger's seminal philosophical work *Sein und Zeit* (Heidegger 1927) has been widely quoted for the past 100 years, predominately in the realm of continental phenomenology, aesthetics and in the various fields of arts research and their contextualisation including dance. In *Sein und Zeit*, Heidegger explores the term 'authenticity' and its opposite: 'inauthenticity'.

Heidegger's thesis of the limits of language and his invocation of a mystical void beyond language were met by a German society that was experiencing economic collapse, hyperinflation and mass unemployment. His persuasive and new use of language, his novel word creations and his idealising notions created an anxious anticipation mixed with charismatic hype in the young generation prior to WW2. "But how will Heidegger lecture if he does not trust in words! Will he come on and be silent? Will he make noises that no one understands?" asks Eleanor in *Hopeful Monsters* (Mosley 1990, p. 115). This novel tells the story of the many interweaving layers of philosophy, politics, science and society at the time that played into the infernal chaos ready to explode with the rise of Nazism. The discovery of Heidegger's *Black Papers* showed how deeply coercive and racially biased some of his thinking had been (Farin & Malpas 2016).

Twenty years later, in the very early postwar period in West-Germany, Horkheimer and Adorno (1947) analysed Heidegger's dualistic notions of authenticity in critical reflections on German society and how it permitted the rise of Nazism. Adorno expanded that, based in the popularity of Heidegger's writing the 'authentic' was exploited as an idealised and absolute notion and in the first half of the 20th century Further Adorno warned that, even in the aftermath of the Holocaust and WW2, German institutions continued to refer to and adopt notions of 'authenticity' that were politically and societally dubious and dangerous.

> in Germany a jargon of authenticity is spoken – even more so, written. Its language is a trademark of societalized chosenness, noble and homey at once – sublanguage as superior language.
>
> (Adorno 1973, p. 3)

Adorno and other philosophers of the Frankfurter Schule of thinking generated and supported the 1960s students' revolution and new developments in the arts. Walter Benjamin (Buck-Morss 1991) and Adorno assessed 'authenticity's' particular notion of a timeless truth. Instead, they regarded truth as bound to history and societal influence and not, as Heidegger had done, as an absolute unchangeable value implied by the term 'authentic'. Heidegger's notions of 'authenticity' in *Sein und Zeit* came again under scrutiny for the way in which they had been used for dangerous idealisation. Heidegger's leanings and his permisssion to let his work be used by the Nazis was fiercely critiqued.

> Throughout his work, Heidegger employed 'authenticity', in the context of existential ontology. Thus in philosophy, he molded that which the authentics strive for less theoretically; and in that way, he won over to his side all those who had some vague reaction to that philosophy. Through him, denominational demands became dispensable. His book acquired its aura by describing the directions of the dark drives of the intelligentsia before 1933 – directions which he described as full of insight, and which he revealed to be solidly coercive.
>
> (Adorno 1973, p. 2)

At a similar time, other critical theorists outside of Germany considered societal contexts as formative to any form of authorship. Barthes (1967) considered society's inscriptions in his seminal essay *Death of the Author*. Barthes is quoted in contemporary dance theory for critiquing the unique authority of the author, meaning the "destruction of the myth of the unitary figure of the master-author" (Lepecki 2006, p. 55). In contemporary theories 'authenticity' continues to be considered a slippery and contested term that implies objectivity, stasis and absolute truth, a Cartesian view. This view appears to be in direct contradiction to Adler's trajectory of non-duality (Adler 2015).

Using the static and potentially judgemental term 'authentic', the possibility of the 'inauthentic' as an opposite to the 'authentic' emerges, with all its pitfalls of judging. However, a witness in Authentic Movement is involved in and influenced by her own being, context and perceptions, whilst a witness observes with an open mind, creating an accepting environment for the mover, one in which she can experience herself as being seen and seeing herself in all and with all imperfections. This premise appears to me to be of prime relevance in a post-modern or post-human world in which the digitalisation of human interactions challenges the ways in which humans as embodied social beings have evolved.

The post-colonial and digitised term 'authentic'

Kemal and Galskell connect the term 'authentic' with notions in the arts and in arts history as being true to a specific historical origin (Kemal & Gaskell 1999). However, in common parlance, the term is nowadays associated with the description and name of all manner of products and services. These mirror the neocolonial attitude and romanticised view that, even in today's world, we may still (or again) find what has been preserved to be original, pure and ... 'authentic'. Seeing the term printed on T-shirts, beer cans and cosmetics is a constant reminder that marketeers are aware of peoples' most deeply seated desires, namely to belong, to have an identity and to have enough. Accordingly, one of the Frankfurt School's arguments against the term 'authentic' was its concomitant use by Western capitalist marketing, a system continually stoking people's dissatisfaction with life. Not new to the 20th or the 21st century, a similar pattern of creating desires can be traced back to marketing campaigns during the industrial revolution and the emergence of modern capitalism, i.e. from early 19th century Britain. Even earlier than that, the term 'authentic' was popular with imports from the British colonies: authentic, British-made goods shipped from the British Isles to the colonies were homey, valued items pacifying homesick emigrants and settlers. Reminding them on foreign shores of their heritage and origins, these goods served as fetishes, symbolic of where their consumers came from and still belonged to. Products made and typical for the cultures of the colonies, in turn, became highly valued, imported articles to Britain, where they became valued as exotic products imbued with the flavours of far away lands successfully conquered and colonised. Human longing and belonging continue to be exploited through the evocative term of the 'authentic'.

Nowadays, the wish to be seen to be 'authentic' is palpably desperate within a homogenised, international, online society and is epitomised by the Selfie and by what I call 'a performance of face'. Personhood, belonging, identity, once defined and supported by a web of family, neighbours, colleagues and friends, surrounding and reflecting an individual, is now a cluster of digital images, tags and links spanning the globe but also skipping the physical presence of persons in actual proximity. Hence, the term 'authentic' has become attached not just to products to make one feel in touch with one's longing but it has been tagged to the individual's digital images of herself: a digital 'authenticity'. 'Authenticity's' flirtation with marketing has increasingly dissociated itself from haptic products and become a commodity of the digitised and virtual world. Prior to society's digitalisation, Adorno stated that

> by denouncing a purely ontological possibility according to his own teaching, Heidegger becomes the advocate of the unfullfilment of life. Like the empty phrase of idealism, authenticity, in projecting its existentialism right from the beginning, sides with want, over and against satisfaction and abundance.
>
> (Adorno 1973, p. 92)

Enquiring into the possible end of an 'authentic' selfhood in a post-modern age Zimmermann (2001) affirms the importance of an ordinary, psychologically intact ego. By ascribing the Heideggerian term 'authentic' and the term 'clearing' to a state of transpersonal becoming, he offers potential understanding of how the mover herself may need to be 'authentic' rather than expect this of her movements. Only by being herself in that sense would she have the ability to sense or know herself to be 'authentic' within the engagement of an activity such as movement.

Applied to Authentic Movement, a witness would have to realise the distinctions between herself and others well before a transpersonal experience, such as empathy expressed in 'I see myself in the other', could be experienced. Perhaps the term 'authentic' cannot be ascribed to an activity but only to a state of inner being. German dance educationalist Artus (1996) states that the term 'authentic' attempts to describe the identity-forming aspects of dance and movement in the practice of Authentic Movement. If the term was not spoilt by capitalist marketing, 'authentic' could perhaps mean an identity-affirming effect, one in which the individual, through practicing Authentic Movement, affirms and strengthens her ego. The ego of a mover has to be intact before the practice can be safely undertaken. Identity is a characteristic of psychological health, one that can withstand the onslaught of images and emotions when engaging artistically or therapeutically with the unconscious. Incidentally, a clear sense of identity can better withstand marketing, digital images and continual digital connectivity.

Towards a new ontology for Authentic Movement: MoverWitness

The aim of Authentic Movement is not to learn how to be more 'authentic' or how to produce 'authentic movements'. The aim is to learn to be oneself in the presence of others and to be embodied and identified with one's body as a living container of mind, organs, muscle and flesh and bones in a digitised world where boundaries between body and machine are increasingly fluid. We are not perfect and any attempt to become 'authentic' so is flawed, leading to deeper suffering of the divide between was is and what could be, between acceptance and desire, between surrender and wishful thinking, and ultimately between oneself and another, or a mover and a witness. So what qualities could help to formulate a phenomenological ontology that incorporates embodiment in all its facets of being, perceiving, moving and speaking?

In the following, I name and briefly sample some of the qualities that I think describe MoverWitness' workings and I shall use this name instead of Authentic Movement for the remainder of this chapter. Qualities overlap, inform each other and closely connect like beads on a necklace, or as movers and witnesses in the group formats of the practice itself. Instead of using nouns that indicate stasis, I experiment with using adjectives and verbs in order to describe these qualities.

Connecting

In the context of a collective body practice format long circle two movers shared an experience of being drawn to each other into a holding embrace reminiscent of that of a mother and her baby. How did this come about? One mover had allowed herself to become regressed to an infant state in which she felt abandoned and alone in a hospital crib. The other mover had felt attracted by the crying of this mover. She had, for her own personal reasons, felt empowered to attend to what became her baby in holding the other mover. In this shared experience, both movers experienced a part of their own personal history. Each one experienced through the other mover a different and more positive outcome than the one originally encountered in their respective lives. Where previously the 'baby-mover' had remained lonely, she was now comforted. Where previously the 'mother-mover' had not been able to attend, she was now happy to be able to do so. The connecting and complementing quality of MoverWitness is one of many examples in which the practice enables opposites to come together, as in past and present; mover and witness; movement and stillness; seeing and being seen; being silent and speaking; individual and group; unconscious and consciousness etc.

Becoming

The above example also serves to exemplify a sense of becoming in the Deleuzian sense where movers and witnesses are altered by what they experience. The dynamic interplay between different movers, the unexpected occurrences and meanings that are shared and constructed develop memories and present insights in an organic sense of becoming. In the practice, there is no objective truth and no objective onlooker. Both mover and witness are subjects and hold their own self-agency and knowledge. There is no right or wrong and various influences between a mover and a witness upon each other are openly acknowledged. Whilst the witness is seated still, she is not static but ready to being moved by what she experiences. Experiences alter all participants, nothing is the same as it was before the engagement with the practice, it is never (or rarely!) boring.

Another experience is that of a group session led by Chodorow in Bologna at The Institute Arte Therapia in 2002. In this group session in which all participants were movers and Chodorow was the sole witness a collective movement ensued within the group of movers. The dynamic of this joint embodiment was so powerful that some movers were temporarily transported into the realm of a collective body-mind. This experience lasted only moments but nevertheless provided a taste of what it means to lose one's boundaries in a state of becoming, similar to collective religious and or tribal ritualistic performative experiences (and I am not promoting here that losing one's boundaries is a good idea!).

Accepting

We are not perfect and any attempt to be so is flawed, leading to deeper suffering of the divide between was is and what could be, between acceptance and desire, between surrender and wishful thinking, and in the practice between a mover and a witness. Whilst being different, a shared commonality at least partially and/or temporarily exists.

> Rather, the practice sets up a non-judgmental framework, which focuses on the relationship between observer and observed, listener and speaker, mover and witness. This relationship is characterised by a welcoming acceptance of whom and what the other is and does. Within this exchange, what may appear authentic to one participant may not seem so to another. This acceptance I understand to be an integral part of the essence and intention of the practice: it enables different perceptions of the same movement event to exist side by side. Methodologically speaking, this is an important assumption and one that I am particularly interested in. It is an epistemological cornerstone, so to speak, a paradigm that bears consequences for how we think about what we do when we engage in the practice.
>
> (Goldhahn 2009a)

Being equal

In Authentic Movement there is no hierarchy of one quality, one movement or one observation being more important than another. MoverWitness is a practice of interaction and relationship that can build a strong sense of belonging and equality between participants. Methodologically speaking, it provides a very elegant, simple score to create an equal playing field for all members of a group. The score sets up the framework for a democratic exchange where each individual contribution can be seen and heard and valued by others. It is a framework that consistently respects individual uniqueness within collective experiences.

In group formats, experiences are shared in movement and in stillness, in being seen, seeing, in not seeing and not being seen, as well as in a speaking ritual dedicated to the present time. In the long circle, everybody begins as a witness to the empty space. Each one can then enter and become a mover in their own time and for a length of time required by their own volition. In breathing circle, the group splits into movers and witnesses with each group taking turns to witness the other group. The speaking ritual follows both formats. The equality between all participants implicit by formats long circle and breathing circle is significant. To be able to both witness and move in equal measure is a sign of an equal participation. The underlying assumptions are:

we are equal; we can see each other; we can hear each other; we can be vulnerable in each others presence; we can choose to respond to each other; we can voice and be heard in our individual experiences.

The outcome of which is: we can trust each other (at least within the boundaries of these circles and their prescribed rules and boundaries). In a sense, these formats create a game or a level playing field. On a political level, we might call such rules essentially democratic.

Sharing

In group formats, a circle of witnesses observes a single mover or a group of movers. Each witness's perspective and perception is different from everybody else's. When speaking and naming these experiences, a multitude of views emerges, with not one of them considered right or wrong. The practice develops a multi-perspective, one that supersedes a singular or singularly, pure or true perspective. Further the idea that movement is solely authored by the mover is antithetical to the influence that movers and witnesses have upon each. When practiced as a group insights gained in MoverWitness weave a complex web of perspectives. Individual viewpoints are immersed into a differentiated collectivity: each one of them is considered necessary for the whole to appear. Akin to contemporaneous concepts in philosophy, influenced by Deleuze and Guattari (1987), I think of all participants' experiences as being inspired and permeated, nourished and contaminated by a multitude of influences; a philosophy that becomes apparent within and through the practice itself.

Permeable

Deleuze and Guattari's ideas of inhabiting a shifting reservoir of involuntary, voluntary, knowable and unknowable, cellular and muscular phenomena, resonate with this. This topography of experiences and of boundaries that mirror both interdependencies and dualities of embodied and mindful experiences demonstrates the ontology of the practice. Again, both long circle and breathing circle, exemplify an underlying ontology that allows participants to experience a philosophy of performance that incorporates movement and stillness, seeing and being seen, democracy, participation and equality. The ontology of the practice appears to be characterized by its complex web of sharing of space, gestures, perceptions, thoughts, breath and particles that inform potential multiple exchanges between a mover and a witness rather than anything static or fixed. Some of these are apparent, visible, haptic and audible, whilst others are hidden from sight, inaudible and can be more difficult to grasp.

Conclusions

The term 'authentic' is critiqued within a historical and philosophical context of continental philosophers, who in the aftermath of WW2 have struggled to come to terms with 'authenticity's' implied notion of perfection and ultimate truth. In contrast, the term Authentic Movement was coined within the American lineage of Starks Whitehouse, Chodorow and Adler (Pallaro 1999) for an evolving and particular type of movement in depth and dance expression using active imagination possibly prompted in its choice of name by Martin's comment on Wigman's historic performance.

Unfortunately, the term harbours the meaning of passing judgment antithetical to the actual practice which is non-judgmental and accepting. Naming movement as 'authentic' creates expectations for a potential realm of perfection and purity that can be seductive and superficial. The seductive potential of the word can be seen in the Heidegerrian, the neocolonial and capitalist uses of the word. Further, the notion of 'authenticity' in its contemporary reading could be seen to be antithetical to the premises of acceptance of being and becoming which are cornerstones of MoverWitness practices. More importantly, and highly pertinent is the attitude of non-judgmental acceptance practiced within MoverWitness: most practitioners and teachers agree that an 'authenticity' of movement, gesture and stillness cannot be a quality per se and that, as such, 'authenticity' cannot be taught or learned.

MoverWitness incorporates the two sides of the coin that are so important to this practice. Movers and witnesses are interdependent in their alternate practices of performing and of perceiving movement, and of following their own individual journeys in movement and in stillness within their own imaginations. Drawing mover and witness together in one name, MoverWitness, back to back so to speak, quite literally illustrates this interconnectivity to newcomers and experienced practitioners alike.

The new name can serve as reminder of what the practice does and how it does it: namely, at least two agents are required to make the practice happen and both these agents contribute to its presence and outcome: it describes both outer conditionality and inner intentions. The name MoverWitness would also reflect a new ontology based on such activities as becoming, stillness and connecting, as well as qualities such as equal, sharing and permeable, all of which are already implied in Adler's primer (2002). Therefore, MoverWitness, instead of betraying or claiming new territory, would help attract newcomers from different disciplines to the practice to study and benefit from the ontological and methodological potentialities of this practice.

References

Adler, J. (1985). Who is the witness? A description of Authentic Movement. (pp i- 23). Self-published copy. Dated November 1985.

Adler, J. (1987). Who is the witness, a description of Authentic Movement. *Contact Quarterly*, 12, no 1, 1987, (pp 20-29).

Adler, J. (1996). The collective body. In Pallaro (Ed.) (1999). *Authentic Movement: Essays by Mary Starks Whitehouse, Janet Adler and Joan Chodorow*. Jessica Kingsley, London, (pp. 190–204).

Adler, J. (2002). *Offering from the conscious body, the Discipline of Authentic Movement*. Inner Traditions, Rochester, Vermont.

Adler, J. (2015). The mandorla and the Discipline of Authentic Movement. *Journal of Dance & Somatic Practices*, 7: 2, (pp. 217–227).

Adorno, T. (1973). *The jargon of authenticity*. Routledge & Kegan Paul, London.

Artus, H. G. (1996). Authentizität, Authentische Bewegung und Tanz., H.-G., Berger, F. R., Rosenberg-Ahlhaus, C. & S. Trautmann-Voigt, S. (Eds.) (1996), *Jahrbuch Tanzforschung*, Heinrichshofen-Bücher, Wilhelmshaven, (pp. 176–194).

Banes, S. (1980). *Terpsichore in Sneakers, Post-modern Dance*. Houghton Mifflin Company, Boston.

Banes, S. (1993). *Democracy's Body, Judson Dance Theatre, 1962–1964*. Duke University Press, Durham and London.

Barthes, R. (1967). The death of the author. *Aspen: the minimalist issue*, 5/6. [Retrieved from http://www.ubu.com/aspen/aspen5and6/threeEssays.html#barthes]

Buck-Morss, S. (1991). *The dialectics of seeing: Walter Benjamin and the Arcades Project*. MIT Press, Cambridge, MA.

Chodorow, J. (1991). *Dance therapy & depth psychology, the moving imagination*. Routledge, London.

Chodorow, J, (2005). Note to Eila Goldhahn, October 2005, Bern.

Deleuze, G., & Guattari, F. (1987). *A thousand plateaus, capitalism and schizophrenia*, University of Minnesota Press, Minneapolis.

Farin, I. & Malpas, J. (ed.) (2016) *Reading Heidegger's Black Notebooks 1931–1941*. MIT Press, Cambridge, Massachusetts.

Goldhahn, E. (2009a). Is authentic a meaningful name for the practice of Authentic Movement? *American Journal of Dance Therapy*. Volume 31, Issue 1, (pp. 53–64).

Goldhahn, E. (2010a). The MoverWitness exchange: interdisciplinary pedagogy and communication tool, towards an embodied and empathetic laboratory. *Poster presentation and workshop, Conference proceedings, Kinesthetic Empathy: Concepts and Contexts, The Watching Dance Project*, Manchester University (22–23 April, 2010).

Goldhahn, E. (2015). Towards a new name and ontology for the Discipline of Authentic Movement. *Journal of Dance and Somatic Practices*, 7: 2, (pp. 273–285).

Heidegger, M. (1927). *Sein und Zeit. Jahrbuch für Philosophie*. In Jahrbuch für Philosophie und phänomenologische Forschung Bd. VIII, ed. Husserl, E.

Horkheimer, M., & Adorno, T. (1947). *Dialektik der Aufklärung, Philosophische Fragmente*. Querido, Amsterdam.

Kemal, S. & Gaskell, I. (1999). Performance and authenticity in the arts. In S. Kemal & I. Gaskell (Eds.) (1999) *Performance and Authenticity*. Cambridge University Press, Cambridge, (pp. 1–12).

Lepecki, A. (2006). *Exhausting dance, performance and the politics of movement*. Routledge, New York.

Martin, J. (1965).*The Dance*. Dance Horizons, New Jersey.

Mosley, N. (1990). *Hopeful Monsters*. Secker & Warburg, London.

O'Donnell Fulkerson, M. (1982). *The move to stillness*. Dartington Theatre Papers, Dartington College of Arts, UK.

Pallaro, P. (ed.) (1999). *Authentic Movement: essays by Mary Starks Whitehouse, Janet Adler and Joan Chodorow*. Jessica Kingsley, London and Philadelphia.

Paxton, S. (1981a). *Contact improvisation*. Steve Paxton in interview with Folkert Bents. June 1981. Dartington Theatre Papers, Dartington College of Arts, UK.

Starks Whitehouse, M. (1958), The Tao of the body. Pallaro, P. (ed.) (1999). *Authentic Movement: essays by Mary Starks-Whitehouse, Janet Adler and Joan Chodorow*. Jessica Kingsley, London and Philadelphia, (pp.41-50).

Starks Whitehouse, M. S. (1963). Physical movement and personality. In Pallaro, P. (ed.). (1999). *Authentic Movement: Essays by Mary Starks Whitehouse, Janet Adler and Joan Chodorow*. Jessica Kingsley, London, (pp. 51–57).

Starks Whitehouse, M. S. (1979). C. G. Jung and dance therapy: two major principles. In Pallaro, P. (Ed.). (1999). *Authentic Movement: Essays by Mary Starks Whitehouse, Janet Adler and Joan Chodorow*. Jessica Kingsley, London, (pp. 73–101).

Zimmermann, M. E. (2001). The end of authentic selfhood in the postmodern age? In Malpass, J. & Wrathall, M. (eds). *Heidegger, Authenticity and modernity. Essays in honour of Hubert L.Dreyfuss*. Vol 1, MIT Press, Cambridge (Massachusetts) & London. (pp.123-148).

Part IV

Authentic Movement's new applications: the MoverWitness

Chapter 9

The MoverWitness: dancers' move to self-agency

Introduction

Shifting seamlessly between poignant gestures and acrobatic feats both classical and contemporary dancers entertain their audiences with the beauty of their highly skilful movement in performance. Their pliability comes at a cost: achieving and maintaining what is considered to be a suitably fit and perfect dancer's body. Being choreographed and performing are highly demanding on body and soul, requiring many hours of work and personal sacrifice to meet those demands. Many training courses and professional companies are aware of these pressures and provide physiotherapy and somatic techniques to ameliorate these effects. However dancers' sense of self-agency and a related politics of dancers' working lives continue to be largely unaddressed (Green 1999, 2002/03, 2004; Hämäläinen 2007; Weber 2011).

Dancers occupy their professional niche with every 'fibre and muscle' of their body and mind as "flexibility, strength and power, cardiovascular fitness, body composition, ethnicity and aesthetics are all factors that contribute to different dance styles in varying degrees" (Bird 2016). Pain, chronic tension, injuries and mental health problems frequently raise their ugly heads in dancers' lives. "90% of dancers had less than 60 minutes at 'rest' at any given time over the course of the working day". (Twitchett, Angioi, Koutedakis, Wyon 2010, p.131). Dance students and graduates are often very young, their bodies and minds not fully matured; this makes them more vulnerable to losing their sense of self and self-agency. Whilst this loss is detrimental to the individual, it is also a loss to dance as a meaningful art form, that depends on its performers thriving.

Challenges

Soili Hämäläinen proposes that

> bodily knowledge has recently been a topic of active debate not only in dance practice and research but also in neuroscience, psychology and philosophy

DOI: 10.4324/9781003222309-13

and that

> bodily knowledge is related and created through perceiving, sensing and feeling.
>
> (Hämäläinen 2007, p. 56)

Being situated at the interface of movement, body and mind the nervous system is the pathway through which sentient beings know their bodily presence and liveness. Bodily knowledge is created primarily through the body in motion and begins its life-long development in everyone's individual genesis in early intrauterine, embryonic movement. Movement and dance can aid the refinement and rejuvenation of bodily knowledge, and is formed in joyous as well as in painful experiences. Authentic Movement's practices teach that bodily knowledge requires conscious awareness of its knower in order to become a useful tool to protect her integrity as a dancer. Being able to name and articulate knowledge verbally assists a consciousness-raising process. When knowledge becomes conscious the knower can own it. Her inner authority can give value to and act upon it (Adler 1987, Olsen 1993, Pallaro 2007).

Body boundaries are one particular aspect of bodily knowledge and they may be understood as a metaphor for the limits and the integrity of a person as expressed in her movements. Julia Buckroyd (2000) states, that many dancers lose their healthy body boundaries during training, no longer clearly knowing what is within and what is without, what belongs to them and what is imposed by others. Dancers may be asked to or aspire to overstretch, overreach or overstep their limits in order to comply with professional training and choreographic demand. Demands of conformity of certain body shapes, sizes and muscle tone or requirements of a specific movement style can distort dancers' perceptions of bodily and psychological boundaries. Without those, a dancer can lose a sense of how far she can go or how close to herself she needs to remain in order to continue to feel whole and herself. She may dismiss where her actual physical and psychological limits are and, with external encouragement and her own wish to achieve, might try to reach beyond towards a perfect goal. Perfection, by its very nature, has a tendency to be always just out of reach and therefore a cause of constant dissatisfaction.

Another challenging experience for dancers can be a sense of fragmentation, a metaphoric splitting into separate, differently valued body parts as Susan Leigh Foster (2012) explains. Dancers, she says, are trained to be technically proficient so that each part can efficiently and accurately respond to demands and movement phrases. It seems to her that in order to convey beauty in movement, a dancer develops a hierachical system of valuation regarding body parts. Repeated experiences of such objectification and fragmentation can challenge the integrity of the dancer and eventually eliminate the trust in her sense of wholeness and bodily knowledge.

Whilst ballet and modern dance techniques contribute to above described issues, problems are reinforced through a widespread societal trend, the keep-fit culture. Machine-based bodybuilding in gyms and the cultural appropriation of elements of yoga, originally a religious Hinduistic discipline, increasingly replace dance techniques and dance improvisation classes. Machine-based work-outs and yoga can build and maintain a body efficiently and quickly but they contribute little to a dancer's sense of herself or to her creativity as an artist. Gyms' machineries evoke images of a modern production line or a military drill suggesting an object-based, external command that can add to a dancer's sense of fragmentation and loss of self-agency. In keeping with pressures of time and space, it may be convenient and seem culturally timely to train and maintain dancers using these methods. Yoga may be deemed politically and philosophically more correct and contemporary than ballet, Graham, Limón and Cunningham dance techniques. But control and supervision come in through the backdoor in a different guise, as disciplines of the exotic and the spiritual. Assuming that yoga must be 'holistic' and Western dance techniques authoritarian, it is tempting to overlook that yoga and some somatic techniques also use control and achievement of posture and external body composition. They can have an equally objectifying and alienating effect on dancers, contributing to a dancer's crumbling sense of self-agency (Green 2004). Dance students and dancers may find themselves no longer within the rigour of ballet or other dance techniques, with their familiar methods of control, but within culturally different, more complex systems of supervision (Green 1999, 2002/03, 2004; Eddy 2002, Hämäläinen 2004). Further, the inclusion of spirituality and meditation can veil elements of 'higher' instances of knowledge or 'wisdom', that continually slip outside of an individual's grasp and achievement. Notwithstanding that any art form can be enriched by experiences outside of its own discipline, there is an epistemological paradox in training dancers increasingly with methods that follow an essentially different aim than the discipline and art form of dance itself.

Whilst many physical and mental challenges originate in the unreflected manner that some methods of dance training are delivered, there are other difficult issues pertaining to dancers' lives. These are the scarcity of job opportunities and, even when working, dancers' economic precarity undoubtedly impacting their stress levels. In the light of critiquing the use of Eastern techniques in training dancers, it seems poignant that many dancers decide to become professional yoga teachers. Primed and prepared by their 'dance training' dancers end up working in the successful and growing health economy instead of in the arts.

Current trainings and professional developments often lack the time and space for dancers to convey and replenish their unique bodily knowing and creative expression. This may be caused by time pressures upon academies, universities and dance companies, but may also be the result of larger economic drivers which determine what is on offer and how bodies are inscribed in order to serve an education system that in turn is determined by economics. A dancer needs time and space for her creativity and her bodily knowledge to flourish.

Moving

Looking for dancing that arises from within a dancer herself and that reinforces her moving knowledge, her creative and emotional imagination and her articulate verbal intelligence, dance educators, somatic practitioners, therapists and researchers such as Olsen (1993), Green (1999; 2004), Hayes (2004, 2006), Hämäläinen (2007), myself (2010) and Payne and Brooks (2018, 2020, 2021a) have sought to adapt elements of Adler's Discipline of Authentic Movement and dance therapy for exoteric use by dance students, dancers, performers and, in the case of Payne and Brooks, more generally for sufferers of medically unexplained symptoms including chronic pain, something which dancers often fall prey to. When practicing Authentic Movement

> we [can] consider dancing for a lifetime, we recognise that we have time to develop our creative and physical resources so that we are not strip-mining our unconscious (using every movement which emerges and putting it on stage) or devouring the vital resources of our body.
>
> (Olsen 1993, p. 49)

Hayes (2004, 2006) researching the beneficial factors of dance therapy on student dancers, found that participants experienced therapeutic benefits from engaging in creative dance within a supportive environment. Hämäläi-nen (2007), who herself experienced Authentic Movement practices, suggests that bodily knowledge could be fostered through methods such as Authentic Movement in dance pedagogy. She states that 'grounding' body experiences enable dance participants to engage more fruitfully with ideas, thoughts, mental images, intuitions and feelings.

To a superficial observer Authentic Movement and the MoverWitness can look like prompted movement improvisations. But they are not. They are neither guided by ideas, concepts, parameters or imagery, nor stimulated by any music. In order to avoid new expectations, such as moving 'authentically' (see preceding Part III) I use the term MoverWitness for working with dancers. MoverWitness practice goes beyond dance improvisation by merit of not suggesting any theme, frame or style. Movers move 'blindly', and any overt mirroring of others is avoided. The practice is pared back to a minimum of what constitutes a relational performative situation: a performer and an observer. No other frame, style or structure is suggested. This provides an open space, enabling dancers to access their own individual movement material. On that basis, dancers get to know and develop their personal, creative movement style whilst maintaining (or regaining) their sense of self-agency, meaning a personhood that is determined from within and resistant to pressures to comply to the without.

Conversely, dance improvisation is educed by many external stimuli: a particular technique, imagery, dance pedagogical or therapeutic style such as in creative dance, mirroring, release dance, contact improvisation or the many improvisations suggested by proponents in this field such as Payne (1990), Miranda Tufnell and Chris Crickmay (1990, 2004). Dance improvisations are informed by a theme and a frame and always reside within a structure and/or a style. They commonly have themes, structures and styles and direct at least one aspect of the improvisers' dancing body-mind within a guiding frame. The aims may be as simple and abstract as suggesting fluidity of movement, use of weight or the imagination of weightlessness, or it may encourage the dancer to keep an anatomical image in mind, such as imagining a line in place of one's spine, when otherwise freely improvising. However, to trained eyes, these improvisations become very easily recognisable as being initiated by a particular direction, school or style of dance. However abstract or imaginative the improvisational tasks, dancers tend to visibly embody the underlying ideas. Even dance therapeutic models of improvisation usually initiate a certain style of movement and dance, one that can be identified as originating in the training of the dance therapist. Groups often conform to ever-so-subtle movement styles, mirroring their teacher and each other even, or especially, in improvisations, as conformity in movement style means to belong to a group.

Liberated from expectations akin to a removal of the obligation of productivity (Instytut Aktors Teatr Laboratorium, 1979), the MoverWitness provides safe time and space for movement per se. The space to move is infused with openness. This way of approaching movement and dance may enable students and dancers to find the needed awareness of their bodily knowledge. This awareness is acquired through spending time listening to oneself and focussing on oneself as the primary source of embodiment. No external teaching or pre-existing know-how has to be taken on board by the dancer. Spontaneous imagery and feelings occur when waiting and moving, creating a feedback loop in dancers to know themselves. They learn to explore their own movement for their own sake, not for the purpose of improving their dance skills and not for choreography or performance. As their inner witness begins to soften they can learn to accept themselves as they are. Adler called the result of this slow and self-directed development of aware bodily knowledge 'mover consciousness' (Adler 2002).

Naturally, any dance training and other learned somatic techniques, machine or yoga-based, becomes apparent as bodies of dancers are inscribed by what they have learned and trained in. However, even a temporary release can open up new horizons that enable what dancers long for; to create and to be seen moving and dancing. Awareness of bodily knowledge corresponds to a growth of personal agency, an ability to set personal boundaries and to know the body and the self as one. Dancers can return 'home' to inhabiting their own body, rather than commanding it as if an object external to themselves; one that needs to undergo a punitive training to perform.

Speaking

According to André Lepecki dance became an autonomous art form by being "dumb and silent" (Lepecki 2006, p. 52). I wonder how can a dancer move and voice her wholeness as a self-determined, speaking artist? What hierarchical and gendered structures need to be disrupted so that dancers can speak (up)?

A common misconception is that Authentic Movement practices simply consist of 'moving and then having a chat about it'. This is wrong, as the movement part, as distinct from improvisation as set out above, is merely the beginning of a more complex learning process enabling the qualities of empathy, non-judgement and non-interpretation through percept language.

> In speaking of an embodied event the mover may describe the movement together with associated feelings, sensations, images, body-felt senses, and thoughts.
>
> (Payne 2003, p. 35).

Bodily knowledge and mover consciousness can flourish when they are verbally processed in witnessing. Verbal exchanges between a mover and a witness are guided by detailed and subtle perceptual, phenomenological rules in order to achieve clear boundaries, respect and containment. They are affirmative to the speaker and the listener as there is no value judgement, and described in detail in Percept language in Chapter 3 of this volume.

The unfolding and seeing of oneself and another in movement and in this verbal exchange is referred to as witnessing and originates from percept language, sometimes referred to as languaging. Participants communicate purely the phenomena of their own, personally authored perceptions. They adopt a phenomenological style of language. This translation of the inherent silence of the movement into a very specific verbal communication creates a dynamic relationship of seeing, being seen, speaking and being heard, in which it is safe to learn from one's own experience and self. It enables being open and vulnerable to a non-judgemental witness. Percept language in the MoverWitness contains, communicates and disentangles complex movement sequences and situations. Whilst words account and analyse much detail of the movement, the particular grammatical use of language weaves and interweaves connections between different levels of experience; a dancer is empowered by learning to speak about her body in movement.

The dancer learns that by developing not just physical memory but verbal recall of movement sequences she speaks about and to her own whole body-self, bridging fragmentation. Taking time to find the words that accept personal movements as they are, dancers can emancipate themselves through their articulate and articulated bodily knowledge. Dance, like all art, is also a political act and depends upon those who can speak out clearly and without fear about their own practice, what they do, how they do it and what it means to them.

As performers, dancers are frequently spoken about and such speaking is often unintentionally judgmental. When talking about dance and performance, those spoken about can easily feel criticised and as if their boundaries are overstepped. According to both Buckroyd (2000) and Hämäläinen (2004), many dance students feel judged, devalued, misunderstood and hurt by an all too common, but insensitive and clumsy criticism relating to their creative dance work. Oberserving dance students' ambivalence between a desire and an anxiety to be seen and to receive feedback, Hämäläinen talks about a 'hunger for feed-back'. She identifies a hypertension that is associated with feedback in dance pedagogy and recommends 'feed-back as dialogue' to defuse this (Hämäläinen 2004).

Relating his own experiences as a dancer, Joshua Monten (2005) describes a choreographer using a 'trick' to cajole her dancers. Accordingly, dancers were asked to change between feelings as if switching programs in digital technologies. This switching was intended to substitute explaining an emotional scene in rehearsal. Switching rapidly between technical feat and conveying emotional expressions is a potentially fragmenting experience for dancers. Being likened to a machine imbues images that sideline a dancer's personhood and creativity. Choreographic 'tricks' such as these sit uncomfortably in a context that foregrounds dancers' integrity.

Most choreography and most dance techniques and somatic classes are delivered via language and this language mirrors their underlying concepts. Thomas Hecht's aptly named essay "Teaching silent bodies" develops a theoretical base in order to examine persisting hierarchical styles of teaching in dance education and elite ballet training. Building on Buckroyd's work he points out that although knowledges exist to work differently, collaborative and explorative ways of working continue to be rarely used in dance education (Hecht 2006). Barthel and Artus (2008) state how critical remarks about dance students' performances in dance education classes discourage dancers' openness and increase their vulnerability. There is an apparent dilemma. Why would dancers be excluded from being encouraged and taught how to articulate their own experiences? Is it because the tradition is that dancers are supposed to do their moves and look good and beautiful and that they are reduced to this function, their mental grasp of what they do considered unimportant? Is it that dance being the domain of girls and women in the past, corporality was considered to outweigh mental ability? I believe that educating articulate dancers is a feminist and a political issue. Percept language is a tool to give witnessing feedback that is non-judgmental and non-interpretive and that empowers its recipient and its speaker alike.

Language plays an important part in handing down hierarchical top-down relationships inscribed in many traditional dance styles and their forms of training. Lepecki comments on choreography's authoritative use of language. He cites Bruce Nauman's early performative pieces in which the artist abides by a set of written and spoken instructions for movement. Following these instructions in physical actions, Nauman leads their sense ad absurdum revealing an authoritarian paradigm inherent in the verbal commands of physical technique and choreography (Lepecki 2006). I have previously described how Nauman and Tino Seghal seem to reference a Foucauldian panopticum in visual performances (Goldhahn 2007).

In choreography, language precedes movement. In MoverWitness, movement precedes language. Where choreography subjects bodies to obediently follow prescription and instruction the MoverWitness's language retrospectively describes a movement that has already taken place. This is not to inscribe it on the dancer's body or make it a repeatable performance like in but to enable the dancer's integration of movement with consciousness. In MoverWitness, language follows movement but it is not secondary in its importance. Conversely, in choreography, language is a means to an end: language aims to bring about movement. It can inspire and instruct dancers on how to move. Movement is the trajectory of choreography's imperative language; it is full of intent for others. Many contemporary improvisations give great scope to dancers, but still instruct and impose specific choreographic intentions and frames via language. The choreographer Rosanna Irvine (2014) uses a soft terminology akin to that of Authentic Movement with phrases such as 'seeing and being seen'. However, typical for choreography's remit, such phrases are combined with grammatically imperative instructions to create scores. In MoverWitness, a dancer is freed from instruction to produce any particular thought or movement. Instead she practices to move and speak only her own bodily knowledge.

Preparing to collaborate

Language, that describes intimate bodily experiences and observations of others' bodies together within a group, demands a high social competence from a leader and teacher so that any connected sensitivities and vulnerabilities of speakers and of the spoken of can be dealt with and held appropriately and safely. The ability and the opportunity to voice what is experienced is essential to mental health and a prerogative to successful learning. Adler (1987) talks about the mover's longing to be seen and considered witnessing, as in languaging, as a way of appropriately responding to this longing. Conversely the complete absence of language can be unmindful of dancers' integrity of body and mind.

Dance therapy improvisations are built around creating self-worth and self-agency within participants. Experiencing oneself as part of a playful, improvising group can in itself promote self-worth. The late dance therapy researcher Jill Hayes (2004; 2006) showed how dancers increased their emotional intelligence in participation in dance movement therapy groups and how this in turn enhanced their sense of identity. Emotional intelligence arises from a knowledge of one's own body and feelings and can foster a deeper understanding and kindness to oneself and others. It is the precursor of empathy. Mirroring, related to the quality of empathy, is a commonly used technique in dance therapy and often takes place in group dance therapy sessions. Here movements and gestures are passed around or imitated, mirrored, when one individual leads and performs. However, a group of participants will largely conform to the movements generated within the group perhaps introduced or amplified by the therapist or group leader. It can be difficult for individuals to break free from the generally agreed movement vocabulary and introduce something entirely new and perhaps more personal or idiosyncratic, something that doesn't feel as though it fits into the group's mould. In professional dance training and practice, dancers are often visually exposed to their own and their peer group or company's reflected mirror images. It can be difficult to know oneself with constant interpersonal mirroring between colleagues, an inner judgemental witness and the ever glaring presence of actual mirrors in the studio.

In MoverWitness, all participants are potential dancers and observers, each one is both, and each one contributes equally. Whilst individual spoken feedback from the teacher/witness is still sought and plays an important role to students, gradually this dependency dissolves into the wealth of a collective group experience. Participants notice that everybody's movement and viewpoint in the group is equally respected and that movements and viewpoints are as different and rich as the multitude of participating witnesses' and movers' backgrounds and experiences. The verbalised dance experiences together with the actual movement experiences create the sum of a multi-faceted image in which individual movers, as well as the collective of dance students, can comfortably exist; there is room and space for each and every experience and expression. Further such learning creates the basis for a collaborative doing together.

Stromsted relates that participants in Authentic Movement practices partake in a non-hierachical collective body (2007). Within this collective top-down and expert relations are dissolved. Movers and witnesses inhabit the same conditions and all of them participate within a 'shared habitat' (Goldhahn 2007); a level playing field. Further, participants in the MoverWitness learn and qualify twofold; after some practice students can learn and practice witnessing themselves. This level of practice enables participants to become proactive within a collectively developed group practice of movement and language. They construct their own experiences themselves without being prone to a judgmental gaze or mirror reflection reminding them to conform to the style or structure of a particular dance style. Thus dancers' fixation with an external, seemingly 'objective' eye upon their bodies' movements may dissolve. Payne explains how participants in Authentic Movement groups may feel closely connected in collective group work:

> Day dreaming is also a non-ego-controlled experience, in which the mind lets go of the separateness normally experienced between the self and other.
> (Payne 2003, p. 34)

Different individuals will take to such work in different ways and at different speeds. As such work is not just about learning facts but about internalising experiences, time is an important factor. The acquisition of bodily knowledge, the maintenance of body boundaries and the healing and knitting back together of a whole-body image and a community of dancers all take time and space. However financial pressures on institutions of artistic training and artistic production means that these can be in short supply.

Conclusions

Whilst the general health benefits of movement, dance and wellbeing are promoted to the general public, little reference about the mental and physical challenges of dance students and professional dancers is made. Whilst dancers are at the forefront of the public image of dance, their plight remains hidden from sight. Complying with a wide range of choreographic and dance training demands can have severe physical and psychological consequences for dancers' wellbeing. Erosion of personal agency can fragment a dancer's integrity of body and mind, her health and creativity. It is these very elements that dance as a unique living art form depends and thrives on and it is essential that dance artists and their gifts are protected. In spite of the proliferation of gyms, yogas and somatic techniques, different improvements to dancers' wellbeing are needed. These must meet and support the inner, psychological process of dancers. Adapting and incorporating particular aspects of Authentic Movement or MoverWitness into the training and continuing professional development of dancers, could in the author's view substantially aid dancers' bodily knowledge, confidence and self-esteem. Three game-changing qualities have been discussed:

- the dancer's awareness of personal bodily knowledge;
- the dancer's ability to communicate through articulate speaking;
- the dancer's experiences of self-agency within a supportive collective as pares inter pares.

In order to teach MoverWitness, a dance pedagogue will need to undergo additional professional training. Such training could create a valuable adjunct skill at dance schools and colleges treating dancers' problems with what they thrive on best: to dance and to move, to be seen and to safely talk about this with peers: freely, outspokenly and equally this could be an antidote to many sins in dance.

Having stated the challenges that face dancers, I note that many contemporary dance artists are already aware of and protect their self-agency carving a niche for themselves, on their own or collaboratively with others. Many contemporary choreographers are respectful to dancers and find new and individually accommodating ways of working collaboratively or, as I describe in the next chapter 10, choreography itself becomes a collaborative endeavour. However,

> As we consider dancing for a lifetime, we recognize that [in Authentic Movement] we have time to develop our creative and physical resources.
>
> (Olsen 1993, p. 49)

References

Adler, J. (1987). Who is the witness, a description of Authentic Movement. *Contact Quarterly* Vol 12, no 1, (pp. 20–29).

Adler, J. (2002). *Offering from the conscious body, the Discipline of Authentic Movement.* Inner Traditions, Rochester, Vermont.

Barthel, G. & Artus, H.-G. (2008). *Vom Tanz zur Choreographie, Gestaltungsprozesse in der Tanzpädagogik.* Athena Verlag, Oberhausen, Germany.

Bird, H. A. (2016). Styles of dance and their demands on the body. *Performing Arts Medicine in Clinical Practice.* Springer, Cham. (pp. 21–37).

Buckroyd, J. (2000). *The Student Dancer – Emotional Aspects of Teaching and Learning of Dancers.* Dance Books, London.

Burckhard, H. and Walsdorf H. (eds.) (2010). *Tanz vermittelt-Tanz vermitteln.* Jahrbuch Tanzforschung Bd. 20, Henschelverlag, Munich.

Eddy, M. H. (2002). Dance and somatic inquiry in studio and community dance programs. *Journal of Dance Education,* Volume 2, No. 4, (pp. 119–127).

Foster, S. L. (2011). *Choreographing empathy, kinesthesia in performance.* Routledge, London.

Foster, S. L. (2012). On Deborah Hay. In *Dance, documents of contemporary art.* Lepecki, A. (ed.), Whitechapel Gallery, The MIT Press, London.

Goldhahn, E. (2007). *Shared habitats, the MoverWitness paradigm.* [Doctoral dissertation, Dartington College of Arts and University of Plymouth, UK].

Green, J. (1999). Somatic authority and the myth of the ideal body in dance education. *Dance Research Journal,* Volume 31, No. 2, (pp. 80–100).

Green, J. (2002/03). Foucault and the training of docile bodies in dance education. *Arts and Learning Research Journal* 19 (1). (pp. 99–124).

Green, J. (2004). The politics and ethics of health in dance education. *The same difference? Ethical and political perspectives on dance.* Rouhiainen, L., Anttila, E., Hämäläinen, S., Löytönen, T. (eds.). Acta Scenica 17, Helsinki, (pp. 65–76).

Green, J. (2007). *Student bodies: dance pedagogy and the soma*, in *Springer International Handbooks of Education*, Volume 16, International Handbook of Research in Arts Education.

Hämäläinen, S. (2004). Ethical issues of evaluation and feedback in a dance class. In *The same difference? Ethical and political perspectives on dance*. Rouhiainen, L., Anttila, E., Hämäläinen, S., Löytönen, T. (eds.). Acta Scenica 17, Helsinki, (pp. 79–106).

Hämäläinen, S. (2007). The meaning of bodily knowledge in a creative dance-making process. In *Ways of Knowing in Dance and Art*. Rouhiainen, L. (ed.). Acta Scenica 19, Helsinki, (pp. 56–78).

Hayes, J. (2004). *The experience of student dancers in higher education in a dance movement therapy group, with reference to choreography and performance.* [Doctoral dissertation]. Roehampton University, London.

Hayes, J. (2006). Reflections on a research process. The experience of student dancers in higher education in a dance movement therapy group with reference to choreography and performance. In Bischof, M., Feest C., Rosiny, C., (eds.). *e_motion, Jahrbuch Tanzforschung*, Bd.16, Lit Verlag, Hamburg. (pp. 173–184).

Hecht, T. (2006). Teaching silent bodies, historical and contemporary perspectives on emotional aspects in ballet education and performing art pedagogy at elite dance conservatoire. In Bischof, M., Feest C., Rosiny, C., (eds.). *e_motion, Jahrbuch Tanzforschung*, Bd.16, Lit Verlag, Hamburg. (pp. 185–204).

Instytut Aktors Teatr Laboratorium (1979). Invitation letter for *Tree of People* E. Goldhahn. 4 July 1979.

Irvine, R. (2014). *Perception frames: choreographic scores for practice and performance.* Middlesex University.

Lepecki, A. (2006). *Exhausting dance, performance and the politics of movement.* Routledge, London.

Monten, J. (2006). Fühlst du, was ich fühle? *e_motion, Jahrbuch Tanzforschung*, Bd.16, Bischof, M., Feest C., Rosiny, C., (eds.), Lit Verlag, Hamburg.

Olsen, A. J. (1993). Being seen, being moved: authentic movement and performance, *Contact Quarterly*, Winter/Spring, Vol 18, no 1, (pp. 46–53).

Pallaro, P. (ed.) (1999). *Authentic Movement: essays by Mary Starks-Whitehouse, Janet Adler and Joan Chodorow.* Jessica Kingsley, London and Philadelphia.

Pallaro, P. (ed.) (2007). *Authentic Movement, moving the body: moving the self, being moved, a collection of essays*, Vol 2, Jessica Kingsley, London.

Payne, H. (1990). *Creative movement & dance in group work*, Winslow Press, UK.

Payne, H. (2003). Authentic Movement, groups and psychotherapy. *Self and Society – Forum for Contemporary Psychology*, Summer 2003, volume 31, number 2, (pp. 32–36).

Payne, H. & Brooks, S. (2018). Different strokes for different folks: The BodyMind Approach as a learning tool for patients with medically unexplained symptoms to self-manage. *Frontiers in Psychology.* (last visited online 20 March 2021).

Payne, H. & Brooks, S. (2020). A qualitative study of the views of patients with medically unexplained symptoms on The BodyMind Approach®: employing embodied methods and arts practices for self-management. *Frontiers in Psychology.*

Payne, H (2021a.) The BodyMind Approach® to support students in higher education: Relationships between student stress, medically unexplained physical symptoms and mental health. *Innovations in Education and Teaching International.*

Rouhiainen, L. (ed.) (2007). *Ways of knowing in dance and art*, Acta Scenica 19, Helsinki.

Stromsted, T. (2007). The Discipline of Authentic Movement as mystical practice: evolving moments in Janet Adler's life and work. Pallaro, P. (ed.) (2007) *Authentic Movement, moving the body, moving the self, being moved: a collection of essays, Vol 2.* Jessica Kingsley, London. (pp. 244–259).

Tufnell, M. & Crickmay, C. (1990). *Body space image: notes towards improvisation and performance.* Dance Books, London.

Tufnell, M. & Crickmay, C. (2004). *A widening field: journeys in body and imagination*, Dance Books, London.

Twitchett, E., Angioi, M., Koutedakis, Y., Wyon, M. (2010). The demands of a working day among female professional ballet dancers. *Journal of Dance Medicine & Science*, Volume 14, No. 4, (pp. 127–132).

Weber, A. (2011). Tanz als Therapie und Therapie für Tänzer: Impulse aus Neurowissenschaft und Psychotherapieforschung. In Birringer, J. & Fenger, J. (eds.) *Dance & Choreomania.* Henschel, Leipzig, (pp. 131–150).

Chapter 10

Collaborative choreography: experimenting with a multi-modal approach

Eila Goldhahn*, Soili Hämäläinen**
and Leena Rouhiainen*** (equal authors)

Introduction

This paper describes the setting up of a new research project at the Performing Arts Research Centre, Theatre Academy, Helsinki, now part of the University of the Arts Helsinki. Its original presentation at the Sibelius Academy in Helsinki as part of the inter-disciplinary conference Embodiment of Authority (2010) served to stimulate discussion, questions and suggestions. The paper traces these early developments of the group.

The Collaborative Choreography Group was formed by Dr. Eila Goldhahn, Dr. Soili Hämäläinen and Dr. Leena Rouhiainen in 2009, in Hamburg, in order to develop an approach to choreographing that surpasses the singular authority of the choreographer and that is uncompromisingly shared, open-ended and emergent in nature. In the case of the Collaborative Choreography Group, it also involves the use of digital media and web-based tools whilst the collaborates were both in close proximity as well as in different geographical settings.

The group first aimed to learn more about collaborative creativity within dance improvisation and choreographing while working as a team. Then its intention was to open the process into a more collective dimension by networking with other arts professionals and social groups. At the conference, the group was physically represented by Leena Rouhiainen and Soili Hämäläinen sharing video footage and commentary on the very early phase of the collaboration. Its purpose was to point out some of the group's guiding principles and to share documentation of the early stage of a collaborative artistic research process that aimed to abdicate/resign from the single authority of the choreographer/art-maker. For the purposes of this publication, the original video footage has been edited down to a shorter summary referred to within the text and can be played alongside the reading on www.sharedhabitat.net.

Background

The joint interests to explore a collaborative form of choreography spring from the contemporaneous approaches to dance-making that

DOI: 10.4324/9781003222309-14

1   underline that choreography is a shared and relational practice of ordering and structuring human movement and its significance in different environments,

2   recommend immediate forms of choreography that take place collaboratively and spontaneously within certain settings of dance and movement improvisations,

3   increasingly utilise digital media and social networking systems as choreographic devices and forums and

4   advocate a social form of choreography and discuss choreographers as frame-makers (Butterworth & Wildschut 2009; Klien et al. 2008).

The latter view relates to choreography as an inter-disciplinary, creative and socio-political act of "setting humans, actions, ideas and thought in relation to one another, to create or reveal order, channel energies, explore dynamics and create conditions for something to happen" (Klien & Valk 2008, pp. 20–21). This is an approach that has inspired the group's thinking. Additionally, in its work, the second view on dance-making relates to pioneering movement therapist Janet Adler's (2002) notion of "Collective Body", a specific concept in the Discipline of Authentic Movement that envisions practices, in which participants spontaneously create group movement.

The Collaborative Choreography Research Group believes that truly collaborative undertakings are considered to be open-ended and involve a shared manner of problem-solving and moving forward with the work (Leinonen 2009). The group also shares general starting points with the so-called devising method. Theatre director Alison Oddey (1994) defines devising performances as a particular form of open-ended collaboration that originates from the interests and interactions of a specific group. It includes working and persevering with the "process (finding the ways and means to share an artistic journey together), collaboration (working with others), multi-vision (integrating various views, beliefs, life experiences, and attitudes to changing world events), and the creation of an artistic product" (Oddey 1994, p. 3; see also Hämäläinen & Rouhiainen 2009). This process demands commitment, sharing responsibilities and interests as well as active initiatives, inputs as well as adaptations from all members of a group.

The Collaborative Choreography Research Group's work is framed by the expertise, skills and interests of its members. Eila Goldhahn's MoverWitness (Goldhahn 2007, 2009a) together with its tool of camera-witnessing offers the group a framework that enables non-directive movement improvisation as well as non-judgmental and participative-observative reception of the danced material. It likewise offers an approach to documenting movement and its verbal reflection. Soili Hämämäläinen's (1999, 2007) interest in the nature of bodily knowledge focuses on perception, sensations and feelings as a source for creative work. In her view bodily knowledge provides the ability to remember, reproduce and create movement. Leena Rouhiainen

(2008, 2010a, 2010b) in turn has explored artistic research as a collaborative and performative venture together with artists working in the field of the performing arts. She is interested in collaborative creativity, the emergent nature of artistic processes and co-relative knowledge production.

When a creative group works together, it creates and operates through mutually built-up routines. These are those that each member brings from previous experiences as well as those which are drawn from new conventions arising from the group working together. These form creative interactions and eventually become what could, after educational theorist Etienne Wenger (1998), be called a community of practice. This is a system of activity amongst participants who share a specific engagement and so develop meanings of what is done together. In this process, the group creates a shared repertoire of skills and thereby ways of solving problems; they create a meaningful understanding of the world and their own practice together (Wenger 1998).

In Wenger's view, participation in a community of practice deals also with a construction of identity, which is known to be an important part of any learning process. To learn is to become someone through active participation (Standal 2009). Embedding artistic learning in a collaborative artistic process allows for learning experiences that are shaped by participation. They are neither completely internalised nor externalised, but located in an ongoing relational process of becoming, namely between the subjectivity of the learner and the negotiative and meaningful constructive activities of the collaborators (Standal 2009). Each group member thus becomes a skilful participant in the collaboration. She expands her artistic knowledge and enhances her capacity to interact artistically (Räsänen 2000). This is what the Collaborative Choreography Research Group aims to accomplish in one of its future work phases.

Creating a new kind of community of practice involves a willingness by all participants to engage in a mutual process as well as openness, trust and sensitivity to each other's acts and reactions. These features relate to feelings of acceptance, reciprocity and safety in human interaction and relationships (Parviainen 2006). They also imply a willingness to follow the initiatives of other group members without a judgmental attitude but with positive curiosity. Approaching creative and collaborative work in this manner allows for flexible integration of individual effort of the group members and a sense of not being alone in the struggle to create. Then group members can indeed co-participate and share the uncertainty of their open-ended endeavours together (Moran & John-Steiner 2004).

Our work-in-progress

Open-ended conversations about our plans and processes are currently our way of realising the above-mentioned goals and principles. These verbal and written communications are likewise supported by studio-based meetings in which we utilise artistic working methods. We have found ourselves brain- and body-storming – the latter being about emotional, sensory and motional observations and expressions of bodily behaviours and acts (Linds & Vettraino 2008).

The method that Eila Goldhahn has introduced to the group is an approach that evolved from elements of the therapeutic practice of The Discipline of Authentic Movement (Adler 2002). It applies improvisatory movement and movement observation tasks from Adler's Discipline of Authentic Movement within the field of artistic research, the MoverWitness (Goldhahn 2007). Camera-witnessing in turn applies the principles of being a witness (in the sense of these practices) into camera-recording of a mover's actions. Put simply, camera-witnessing utilises a single perspective and applies a non-judgmental attitude and positive regard towards the seen. This can be movers improvising or other subjects and/or objects. What makes it distinctive is the humane and soft gaze that is applied whilst using a camera (Goldhahn 2007).

The above-mentioned methods appear to support the emergence of creative understanding of both the groups' shared processes and each individual's experiences and acts. In collective body formats in MoverWitness, all participants are simultaneously potential witnesses and movers. They can respond spontaneously to the group by becoming movers and decide when to withdraw from moving to be witnesses to the group. Each mover, in pursuit of their own pathway and movement pattern that is 'correct' to them at any given moment in time, is also open to the collective soundscape and kinaesthetic landscape, constantly responding and contributing to collective needs as they unfold. Participants are active members of a constantly evolving collective movement-image (Goldhahn 2007).

Further articulation and understanding of the movement practice emerges when movers and witnesses verbally exchange their perceptions. Then they speak about their experiences and may discover the 'shared habitats' or moments in which movement and witnessing experiences meet. The careful linguistic separation and clarification of individual experience frequently reveal similarities, interdependencies and differences between participants. This happens also when the filmed material is viewed. It allows participants to observe a shared event from new perspectives. We find shared descriptive writing to do this, as well. All these measures allow for a dynamic intertwinement of different experiences. They support the emergence of socially shared understanding of the group's embodied undertakings. The revelations of varied realities conclude with a shared commonality between all participants. In this sense participants' experiences are inspired and permeated, nourished and contaminated by a multitude of influences (Goldhahn 2007).

The Workshops

So far we have met and worked together in two short workshops. The first was in Helsinki at the Theatre Academy, the second was held partly outdoors on the island of Pettu in Southern Finland as well as in Merihaka and the Hanasaari power plant in Helsinki in addition to the studios of the Theatre Academy. In the midst of the second workshop we wrote the following summary of what we had done so far:

Meeting at Theatre Academy in Helsinki in February 2010

> Following a larger seminar for staff and research students in her applied methods Eila led sessions for the new research group. In these the group improvised undirected movement within the MoverWitness which allowed the group to get to know each other in an embodied and artistic way. The group also practiced camera-witnessing in order to both observe, share and document these processes. The learning processes were both methodological, artistic and personal and opened up a new platform of shared experience.

Meeting in Pettu and at Theatre Academy in Helsinki in August 2010

> Soili and Leena demonstrated how they worked together in their previous artistic collaboration that produced two solo dance performances. In the studio they led movement exercises that consisted of breathing, opening the body through internal stretch, weight release, hiding and revealing body parts as well as working with spatial parameters. All three participants also moved together. Returning to discuss the nature of the collaboration the group found its meeting point to be in the fact that the emergent process would reveal the goals, working methods and contents of the group. Process oriented and open-ended group work allows for changes in focus according to the life, interests and developments of the group and can be conceived of as a radical approach to co-operation. For the group it was an exciting approach allowing freedom and fostering creativity through mutual learning and inclusion. By its very nature this collaboration is about an embodied process: brainstorming and body-storming to find answers.

Whilst exploring how to continue the process of working together the group watched video footage produced by Eila and Soili on Pettu island. Seeing dance improvisation in the beauty of a landscape with rocks and sea triggered the idea of going out into an urban environment to work within a very different setting. Going to an urban shore of Merihaka, a high-rise dwelling area next to the Theatre Academy, the group became fascinated by the massive black coal heap of the Hanasaari power plant both as a visual inspiration and as a possible metaphor for the work itself.

The video footage so far produced gives an example of camera-witnessing in the first section where Leena and Soili are seen improvising with their eyes closed in a studio at the Theatre Academy. The camera-witness, Eila, is still except for small movements where she adjusts the frame to the movers altering their positions in the space. This is similar to turning one's head whilst remaining in one place when witnessing without a camera or when being part of a seated audience in a performance. It is different and more personal to a usually filmed document of performance where a more objective perspective is both assumed and offered.

In the following section filming and movement take place outdoors alternately by Eila and Soili. Whilst the floating stage is a familiar space to Soili, the landscape and the beach are unfamiliar to Eila. This difference appears to be apparent in their movement.

A long, hand-held shot of the moonlight on the water was added into the group's footage and stands in for the pausing for reflection and the not-knowing at the beginning of a research project.

The jointly, improvised movement exploration of the floating stage opposite the big black coal heap within the city uses instead a fixed tripod-mounted camera that allows all three collaborators to move together. This setup produced less-animate images than the ones that are hand-held and camera-witnessed but has perhaps more interesting dynamics as three women move on a small and constantly shifting 'stage'. Here the video footage provides a visually more colourful, animated documentation of the tacit processes involved in the research process.

Conclusions

Regarding the overall manner in which the group worked, it was noticeable that, within the open processes, we were able to allow for new happenings in the group to trigger further action. All members were simultaneously reflexive of and contributing to the themes that were dealt with and addressed. The group continually questioned, for example, the content of the video footage: what was it addressing and what was it for. But the group also asked what happens when one works according to collaborative, spontaneous and intuitive choreographic decisions: where does this process lead, and in fact if it leads anywhere. What kind of collective embodiment was this group creating by sharing the present moment and locations in moving, filming, discussing and writing as well as working through web-based media across geographical distance and different temporal moments?

Whilst relinquishing individual, artistic authority, the group has begun its process of questioning how a collaborative process evolves as a mode of movement exploration, dance-making and producing digital visual and written material. It is in the process of exploring how the group's emergent collaborative approach and social aesthetics are produced and mediated by the three collaborators in their different ways. What will be additionally probed is, how can this process be understood as performative artistic research? The negotiations between form and content, method and outcome become the precipitous edge on which our cooperation in collaborative choreography hinges.

References

Adler, J. (2002). *Offering from the conscious body, the Discipline of Authentic Movement.* Inner Traditions, Rochester, Vermont.

Butterworth, J. and Wildschut, L. (2009). *Contemporary choreography, a critical reader.* Routledge, London.

Goldhahn, E. (2007). *Shared habitats, the MoverWitness paradigm.* [Doctoral dissertation, Dartington College of Arts and of Plymouth, UK].

Goldhahn, E. (2009a). Is authentic a meaningful name for the practice of Authentic Movement? *American Journal of Dance Therapy.* Volume 31, Issue 1, (pp. 53–64).

Hämäläinen, S. (1999). *Koreografian opetus- ja oppimisprosesseista – kaksi opetusmallia oman liikkeen löytämiseksi ja muotoamiseksi [Teaching and Learning Processes in Composition – Two approaches to find one's own movement].* Teatterikorkeakoulu, Vantaa, Acta Scenica 4.

Hämäläinen, S. (2007). The meaning of bodily knowledge in a creative dance-making process. Ways of Knowing in dance and art. Rouhiainen, L. (ed.). Acta Scenica 19, Helsinki. [www.teak.fi/Tutkimus/Tutkimushankkeet].

Hämäläinen, S. and Rouhiainen, L. (2009). A somatic and collaborative approach to dance-making. *Dance Movement Mobility Proceedings*, 9th International Nofod Conference. Leena Rouhiainen ed. (pp. 186–193). University of Tampere, Department of Music Anthropology.

Klien. M. et. al. eds. (2008). *Framemakers: choreography as an aesthetics of change.* Daghda Dance Company Ltd. Limeric, Ireland.

Klien, M. & Valk, S. (2008). Choreography as an aesthetics of change. *Framemakers: Choreography as an Aesthetics of Change.* Michael Klien et. al. eds. (pp. 20–25). Daghda Dance Company Ltd., Limeric, Ireland.

Leinonen, T. (2009). Different forms of collaboration in learning. FLOSSE Posse, Free, Libre and Open Source Software in Education. http://flosse.dicole.org/?item=different-forms-of-collaboration-in-learning [last visited 30 May 2009].

Linds, W. & Vettraino, E. (2008). Collective imagining: collaborative story telling through image theater. *Forum: Qualitative Social Research*, Volume 9/2, Art. 56.

Moran, S. & John-Steiner, V. (2004). How collaboration in creative work impacts identity and motivation. Dorothy Miell & Karen Littleton (eds.) *Collaborative creativity: Contemporary perspectives* (pp. 11–25). Free Association Books, London.

Oddey, A. (1994). *Devising Theatre. A Practical and Theoretical Handbook.* Routledge, London.

Parviainen, J. (2006). Kollektiivinen tiedon rakentaminen asiantuntija työssä [Collective Knowledge Construction in Expert Work]. *Kollektiivinen asiantuntijuus*

[Collective expertise]. Jaana Parviainen ed. (pp. 155–187). Tampere University Press, Tampere.

Räsänen, M. (2000). *Sillanrakentajat. Kokemuksellinen taiteen ymmärtäminen [Bridge Builders. Understanding Experiential Art]*. Taideteollinen korkeakoulu, Helsinki.

Rouhiainen, L. (2008). Artistic research and collaboration. *Nordic Theatre Studies*, Volume 20, (pp. 51–60).

Rouhiainen, L. (2010a). A mono-trilogy on a collaborative process in the performing arts. John Freeman (ed.) *Blood, Sweat & Theory, Research Through Practice in Performance* (pp. 139–150). Libri Publishing, UK.

Rouhiainen, L. (2010b). Dancing emplacement in an installation entitled *Passage*. Pape, S. (ed.) *Norsk Dansforskning* (pp.15–36). Tapir Akademisk Forlag, Trondheim.

Standal, Ø. (2009). *Relations of meaning. A phenomenologically oriented case study of learning bodies in rehabilitation context*. Dissertation from the Norwegian School of Sport Sciences.

Wenger, E. (1998). *Communities of practice. Learning, meaning, and identity*. Cambridge University Press, Cambridge.

Chapter 11

Being seen digitally: exploring macro- and micro-perspectives

Introduction

Some ideas in this chapter were originally presented at the Conference of the European Association for Dance Therapy in Athens (2018) and served to stimulate discussion and questions. This edited essay was subsequently published in *Body, Movement and Dance in Psychotherapy* in 2021.

Working digitally, online and on-screen, occupies an increasing amount of time in dance therapy and in other arts and psychotherapy practitioners' working lives. Time in the physical presence of clients and students is constantly decreasing. Prior to the Coronavirus crisis, only a few practitioners thought about the impact that digitally mediated sessions (instead of direct personal contact) might have on their work with clients. Since then, reflections and insight into how digital communications work, their politics and ethics, and their impact on mental health and somatic therapies, teaching and supervision practices have emerged. Reflecting on the influence of macro drivers this chapter suggests practical steps to make improvements on the micro-level of digitally offered therapies. I suggest that aspects and qualities of witnessing, as introduced by Adler in the Discipline of Authentic Movement (Adler 2002) and used in camera-witnessing in the MoverWitness (Goldhahn 2007), may be adapted to aid online work.

Roots of this work

Adler's article Who is the Witness (1987) explains the relationship between a mover and a witness. Mover and witness are inextricably connected in their influence upon each other's experiences and it is this connectivity that provides the ground for a profound healing presence in being seen and heard. This takes place in the actual physical and perceptual presence of participants who share the same space and time; they are together. In my arts-led PhD research, I explored film and other visual arts in relationship to movers and witnesses (Goldhahn 2007). I was particularly interested in how the Discipline of Authentic Movement's underlying philosophies and workings

DOI: 10.4324/9781003222309-15

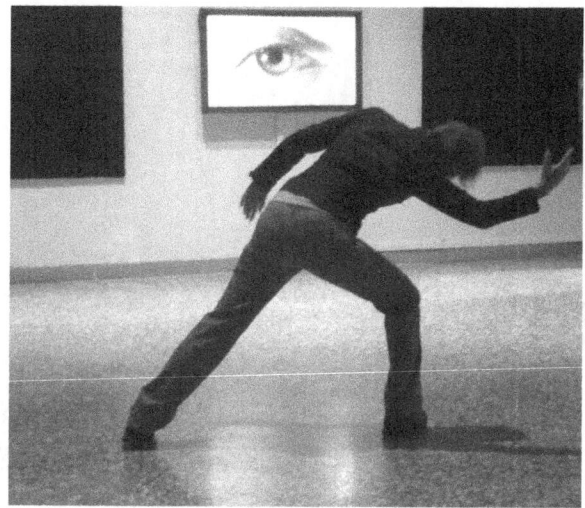

Figure 11.1 Eila Goldhahn dancing in front of artist Lorenzo Hemmer's installation at Venice Bienale. Photo: Stuart Young (2009)

could provide a transferable method, the MoverWitness. I found that by applying witnessing skills to my practice of filmmaking, my empathetic and aesthetic experiences became visible to others in the footage. Participants found a coherence between their own experiences as movers and what they saw in my footage. One person stated that "I was surprised that I was neither shocked nor offended by seeing myself moving on film". And another shared that "The footage bears witness to your witnessing of us, Eila, albeit silently". As my work developed over several projects, I came to use the term camera-witnessing.

It applies the same principles as personal, silent witnessing namely observing with interest, positive regard and the intention to not judge or categorise the seen. Using this approach I have also made films applying MoverWitness practices and shown these as art installations in public arts venues (Figure 11.2).

The following principles of camera-witnessing crystallised as being particularly useful when working with others. They form part of an evolving way of working with film and other digital media that foregrounds ethical considerations.

Camera-witnessing

1 Preparing a safe space

In addition to confidentiality and privacy, as required in all therapeutic settings, a safe space involves openness about the presence and purpose of

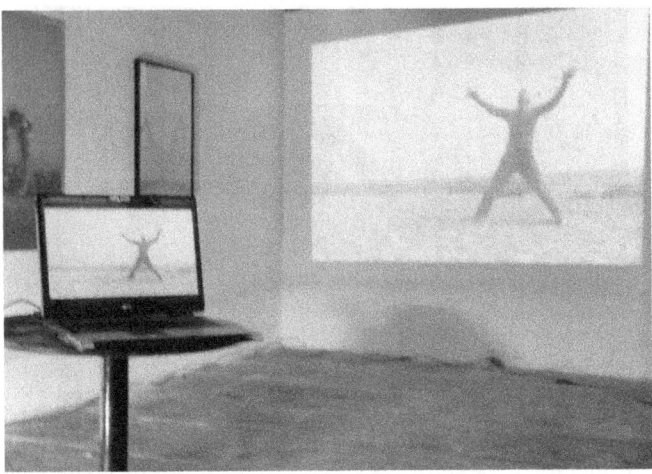

Figure 11.2 Slapton beach movers, 2-screen digital film installation at the exhibition Dark Energy, Plymouth. Artist: Eila Goldhahn, 2017

the camera and the filming. A camera or another recording device, a laptop, is akin to another entity that needs to be known in order to be consciously accepted. For example, the camera can be handled by participants themselves and the purpose of the filming can be openly explained and discussed.

2 Positioning

As in the Discipline of Authentic Movement, also a witness with a camera does not move around the room but stays in the same place. This allows a mover to always know where the witness is and to move into the witness's blind spot if there is a need not to be seen. I use only one fixed, seated position so my perspective remains entirely predictable to the movers whilst they have their eyes shut.

3 Witnessing with a camera

As a camera-witness, I remain seated and quietly positioned whilst able to move forward or back and yield. My neck and head are able to turn, to rise and to follow. Whenever I can, I look above my camera's viewfinder to be in direct contact with my movers. Like this, I am able to use tilts, turns and slow zooms similar to the way I observe movers without a camera. The subtle movements of my upper body and the focussing of my eyes are reflected in the footage that I take.

4 Following one's inner witness

A witness's gaze is typically mindful of her own inner witness and rooted in the consciousness of her own body. She is quiet and alert and follows the mover with an open, non-judgemental gaze. As a camera-witness, I attend to my own body and, by becoming conscious of my somatic and feeling responses, these become apparent in the resulting film footage. As in witnessing, I allow my body to be subjectively tuned into the moment of the mover's presence. For example, my own rhythm of breathing mirrors my emotional responses and this too can be subtly visible in the footage.

5 Vetting the footage

As in the Discipline of Authentic Movement, also in the MoverWitness the mover is the explicit expert and authority of their own movement material. My work with the camera is based on being a silent witness and movers are ultimately in charge of their movement material. This is similar to being a witness who only responds to the mover's explicit ask for witnessing in response to what the mover has recalled already herself. After the live movement and camera-witnessing session is digested and integrated, movers are invited to see and vet the film footage. If someone wants to not see it or wants to exclude something about themselves, I accept this and edit accordingly. The mover's authority always takes precedence over my own vision for a film.

Digital technology in psychotherapy and somatic practices

As camera-witnessing became my practice for filmmaking it also grew into my approach for digitally conducted online sessions. However, when thinking about online encounters and transferring camera-witnessing to screen relationships, I wanted to find out more about the larger world of techno-politics. Realising that unknown parameters of the digital world have an impact on work in dance therapy and somatics I decided to explore not just the microcosm of sessional work but also some of the macro perspectives on digital technology. I sensed that with increased use of digital communication, complete ignorance of its workings can lead to powerful illusions. As therapists we know that taking things for granted without reflection and knowledge can be counterproductive to our work with clients and students. I felt that without knowing the context and impact of digital tools, it might be impossible to fruitfully examine what can be helpful to our field. One of the most common and questionable misconceptions regarding digital communications I found to be the idea of 'presence'.

The world's economies are based on digital communications that are applied to all aspects of human life. This holds true for the field of humanities and psychotherapies, namely those areas where in the past actual bodily human presence was considered an essential prerogative, its conditio sine qua non. This understanding appears to no longer be held. Why is this so?

The digital sharing economy is a platform that now affects the work of most therapy practitioners and will increasingly do so. Whilst many consider working in this way less than perfect, others embrace this new way of working enthusiastically. How can we transfer our therapeutic foundations and ethics to mediated sessions? And how can bodily presence approach a digital 'presence' mindfully and holistically? Is that possible?

One of my students of The Discipline of Authentic Movement wrote to me: "The economic convenience for me as a practitioner, to be able to not need to rent space for Skype sessions is an enormous advantage at this stage where, frankly, I need paid session hours over idealised session hours". It is interesting that he considers bodily presence with his own clients to be an ideal, rather than a condition for his work. He is not alone in the field. It is clear that to many practitioners, using digital communications for sessional work makes practical and, importantly, economic sense.

To many practitioners, being together in physical space and time has become a precious and rare commodity. Embodied presence and real life encounters between movers and witnesses, therapists and clients have become a luxury. They are reserved to occasional, sometimes annual, retreats and training whilst most of the therapeutic, supervisory, mentoring or training encounters take place online. This is by email, online study modules and reading, and by using Skype, Zoom and similar applications. This technology has provided substantial advantages to reach dance therapy clients and trainees in countries where such therapeutic practices were formerly unknown. What is lost in these translations? What new understanding do we need to be mindful and skilful of in the practice of digitally mediated sessions if these are unavoidable for most practitioners?

The economics of digital communications are based on speed and ubiquitousness, qualities that are considered to be positive. Digital media enable practitioners to reach out to an international community of potential clients, students and supervisees around the clock. Speed, and availability to speed, equals money in economic terms and is the driver of technological development. It has driven the imminent shift from 4G to 5G networks and will soon be superseded by holographic mediation in turn. The difference between 4G and 5G technology is the speed of transmission of data. 5G decreases the current latency, the time lag in digital communications, and increases users' perception of real-time and real presence when online. Holography, in turn, is going to create a three-dimensional experience and will be yet a step closer to so-called 'presence' in media technology.

4G communications are asynchronous with a latency (time lag) of 10 or more milliseconds. This is small yet perceptible. It is latency that creates a sense of distance and disruption to mediated communications in 4G. Participants feel as though they have to pause and wait during communications and that they do not really connect and communicate at times because of this lag. This makes bodily attunement, such as joining each others rhythm of breathing, difficult.

Human senses and social interactions evolved and adapted to function optimally in the presence of another body equipped with these same senses. The evolutionary function of innate mirror neurons is based on individuals being in each other's presence, of having eye contact, of being in earshot, of joining each other's rhythm of breathing, to read and emphasise with facial expressions and gestures. There is no evolutionary facility to effectively adapt to and deal with a time lag between human communicators. Therefore, feelings of understanding and empathising with each other can be said to be lost in the translation of the digital data between one screen and another. Communicators often show signs of tiredness after a shorter period of time compared to being in each other's presence, when focus and attention can be held for longer periods of time. In part this is due to the distortions of image and sound and the nervous system having to fill in the gaps of poor visual and auditory signals. Tensions normally eased during a therapeutic session may persist due to this strain on perceptions.

Further media psychologist Jeremy Bailenson identified close up screen-based visuality, mental overload, self-mirroring and lack of movement as the major contributing factors to screen fatigue (Bailenson 2021).

5G is considered 'real-time' internet and is therefore desirable. It will reduce latency to one millisecond, a time lag so small that it is imperceptible to the human nervous system. 5G is considered a great improvement in digital communications as it increases the felt sense of individuals' connectivity. 5G will also improve the resolution of streamed video images making the response to physical expression more possible. It will mediate the experiences of seeing online and on-screen with increased visual resolution and depth of field. This means that the digital images that we see of each other are going to appear more real and more like real-time, furthering the illusion of providing real contact and presence with another person. This appears to be good news for therapists and psychotherapists working with the body, movement and somatics. 5G will create a more powerful illusion of 'presence' than 4G is able to. However it will not replace the human need for body to body presence. This was shown by the increase in mental health issues during the pandemic's lockdowns when the increase of digital meetings replacing real live contact first dramatically increased.

The spread of Western somatic therapies and dance therapy into countries such as China and India has been enabled by the use of digital technologies Whilst these exchanges have been creating new insights and culturally adept ways of practicing, the internet has also enabled the West to spawn its ideas about culture, standards of living and an imagined white racial supremacy.

Further, the use of the internet is connected to a worldwide increase in energy consumption. Mega hubs fuel large servers necessary to provide the computing power to enable the world wide web to function. Being ubiquitously available around the clock, digital technology and economy consume energy to work. During the lockdown, the increased use of the internet led to increased domestic energy consumption whilst energy consuming air travel decreased. Subsequently media psychologist Jeremy Bailenson was able to show that less than 10% of energy is required for video conferencing than for an in-person meeting (Bailenson 2021).

However there are also less measurable, societal consequences of people encountering each other less frequently. Sociologist Norbert Elias proposed that, as our bodies less frequently approach, move towards, gather and move around and away from each other, the opportunity for democratic society diminishes. Elias described societies as figurations of bodies that move similar to those in a societal dance. He argued that democratic society is largely a physical, corporal process that needs practising just in that way, like a ritual (Elias 1994, v. Randow 2020). What happens when we no longer dance with each other? How do we as therapists feel after a mediated session or after a session with our client or student present? What happens and is denied us? What happens to our desire and the souciance of bodies and minds seeking to connect with each other in therapy, training and somatic practice? Whilst pertaining to be an economic blessing, there are personal, political and ecological costs to mediated communications.

Do you see me? Do you hear me?

The title of this section uses phrases from the Discipline of Authentic Movement (Adler 2002). They are the essential, urgent and prime questions a mover may ask her witness. 'Yes, I see you', replied with sincerity can be profoundly affirming to the mover. When we engage in online therapy or training sessions, this same phrase is often spoken with a different purpose. We actually mean: is the technology between us working? Can we see a mediated image of each other on each other's screens?

What was originally meant by Adler and her students to be a deeply affirmative echo of physical presence and meaningful understanding within an intimate sharing of private space and time, means something very different in digital communications. The different meanings can evoke a bizarre echo of the former and become, completely unintentionally, confusing. Taking time to clarify what it is we mean, namely two people gazing at each other on two screens across a vast distance, we can practice consciousness even before we begin our actual mindful practice. The absence of bodily presence and the separation of therapists and clients or teachers and students in different spaces imposes a layer of alienation requiring an alert, discerning consciousness and communication style, that can at least ameliorate these effects.

In digital communications, nobody actually does 'see' or 'hear' each other but the interpersonal contact, whether perceptibly lagging in time or imperceptibly brought near to perfection as in 5G, is technologically mediated via super-fast digital signals and unscrambled for its recipients. Meanwhile, each participant remains solely in a different time and space. The word digital refers to signals and data that are expressed as series of the digits 0 and 1, so-called binary data. They are typically expressed in values of voltage or magnetic polarisation. Computer technology uses these binary, digital data in order to process and communicate information fast across vast distances. When in digital communications to say 'I see you' it indicates that pixels on a screen have formed into the digital recognisable image of another person or yourself. 'I hear you' in turn means that the participants' voices are transmitted via microphones and digital inscriptions and then unwound by recipients' computer soft- and hardware into audible sound bites. The perfect illusion that will be created by 5G and by holography requires participants to be even more conscious of their site in time and space, as there will be ever less to remind us that the other person is not in our actual presence. I believe that it is fundamental to our work to foster a conscious relationship that continues to distinguish between mediated and unmediated, direct presence and digital experience.

Whilst time spent in front of two screens sometimes thousands of miles apart in different time zones may be considered shared time, it does not constitute shared space. Shared space enables a direct experience of the other person, the potentiality of haptic contact, touch, the presence of smell, the presence of atmosphere of shared air and breath, the potential of bacteria and virus being present, the potential of intermingling and permeation of shared habitats (Goldhahn 2007). In front of a screen I cannot touch, smell or move with the other. I am physically removed from the other. This raises therapeutic questions such as the safety in mediated therapeutic practice. What happens when a client disintegrates and finds themselves essentially alone? What if we need to hold, support the client with our body or simply breathe with them?

Gillian Isaac Russell's aptly named book *Screen Relations* (Isaacs Russell 2015) offers an in-depth analysis of the *Limits of Computer-Mediated Psychoanalysis and Psychotherapy*. Isaacs Russell begins from the premise, adopted by many psychoanalysts using the internet for client contact, that psychoanalysis is two minds talking to each other (as opposed to two bodies 'talking' to each other!). She critically examines current practice and offers some improvements. Her main message calls for conscious handling of the medium. She also sets out how body-to-body presence is a prerogative to building trust and relationship between analyst and analysand. Her critical arguments echo mine. She urges us "not to automatically adjust our perceptions to fit the limitations of the tools" (Isaacs Russell 2015, p. 156) and encourages us to create residual trust by building a face to face relationship that is based on body-to-body presence prior to engaging in online sessions with a client (Isaacs Russell 2015).

Ethical values are reflected within the therapeutic or supervisory space that we offer and I suggest that we extend that responsibility and awareness to the medium we employ. I am proposing a methodological shift that embraces the medium, making the medium part of the space we create.

Some suggestions for online work

The culture of the self-styled selfie is often criticised by people seeking 'authenticity' but for the purpose of 'being seen digitally', it might be helpful for therapists and clients to think as being engaged in imagining and creating moving selfies of themselves. When we position ourselves in front of our computer or laptop cameras, we are creating an image of ourselves. When we click the camera icon, we begin to film ourselves and permit this film to be transmitted to another in an instant.

By acknowledging and admitting that we are creating moving selfies for each other, we might bring greater self-reflection and honesty into our digital encounters. To talk about and acknowledge that we are filming ourselves for another can also affirm a sense of self-agency. This sense of being in control aids the production and projection of a self-image. A conscious and creative self-agency helps to bridge the inescapable void in digital encounters and can also be an expressed therapeutic aim. Clients may explore how and why a particular image of themselves is created, neglected or co-created together with the therapist/teacher.

The student/mover/client remains on her own in her own space in digitally-mediated sessions. It takes leaps of imagination to think and believe in being truly witnessed in this manner. I believe that some clients' sense of alienation cannot be bridged but might deepen into despair by this way of practicing, which will require very careful handling. Being seen digitally requires an increased amount of circumspection, preparation, trust and imagination and sensitive consideration as to what groups of clients this can be responsibly offered to.

The need to be close is mirrored in participants' tendency to move ever more to their screens in a seemingly desperate attempt to feel intimacy. Conversely Bailenson identified screen proximity as a disturbing factor, as artificially close proximity is usually reserved for intimate encounters (Bailenson 2021), and not for therapeutic encounters or meetings.

The ethics of witnessing and camera-witnessing, as shared earlier in this article, can be thoughtfully adapted for creating a safer, therapeutic space for our online encounters in dance therapy and somatic practice. The following pragmatic guidance might be helpful to being seen and heard more fully when online.

Choose or create a space in front of a day-lit window or an artificial light source. This aids your computer camera to film you. Avoid back or ceiling lighting as it will detract from what your client/student will want to see namely your face and eyes.

Have your camera/laptop in front of you on top of a small table or a pile of books. The camera of your device has to be the height of your head to give a sense of equality in the digitally transmitted encounter.

Avoid tilting the computer screen with its in-built camera back in order to capture you. This leads to your face being shown from below. The recipient will look up at you, a position suggesting childlike inferiority.

For somatic movement work in which you too plan to move, map out a space behind yourself. Due to the way lenses work the optics fan out, giving a perspective of three-dimensional space. Mark this trapeze-shaped space with rolled-up blankets.

Get ready for your session: have a couple of quiet minutes before dialling in with each other.

Use only an auditory signal to begin with and check that you can clearly hear each other. Adjust the volume/microphone. Hearing each other is the basis for visual contact as it is easier to accept. Once good auditory contact is established, use this to check-in and tune in with each other.

When you can hear each other well and feel that you have made contact with each other, check that you are ready to switch on the visual video signal.

Adjust the angle of the computer camera so that you feel comfortable with the image that is projected of yourself.

Begin to make visual contact with the other person. Give each other time to describe: Can you see me on your screen? What is the image of myself like? If applicable check that each other's marked movement space works well for the other person and make adjustments as necessary.

Acknowledge you are meeting online and that you might get tired of each other's digitally transmitted words and images, because being seen and heard digitally is much harder than being together in one space. Allow sessions to be shorter than they would be in each other's presence to take account of this fact. Share your practical steps with your student/client/partner. They will find it useful to be on the same page as you.

When introducing my preparations to a dance therapy colleague, she stated: "I was looking for ways to improve my online encounters with clients. Now I feel that I have a practical set of parameters to enable me to do this". Another peer echoed this, saying that she had felt inhibited taking on students for online sessions. She felt that she needed to practice my suggested ideas and steps to offer online sessions confidently. She wanted to make these part of her skill-set.

Conclusions

When a digital device is used, this becomes an integral part of the therapeutic container, process and practice itself. The lack of shared bodily presence is always palpable in these encounters, yet, as we are driven by necessity, it is tempting to blend these out. Whilst leaps of imagination are useful in bridging the gaps, the need to be seen and heard in the bodily presence of another, remains. As also in mediated presence the mover/client remains the expert of themselves, a moving selfie may be seen as a personal expression of just that. Verbal checking-in and witnessing become an important verification of what may or may not have been seen in digital translation. Meanwhile, we need to remember that we continue to long to be seen and heard in the physical presence by another in shared space and time.

References

Adler, J. (1987). Who is the witness, a description of Authentic Movement. *Contact Quarterly,* 12, no 1, 1987, (pp. 20–29).

Adler, J. (2002). *Offering from the conscious body, the Discipline of Authentic Movement.* Rochester, Vermont, Inner Traditions.

Bailenson, J. N. (2021). Nonverbal overload: a theoretical argument for the causes of Zoom fatigue. *Technology, Mind, and Behavior,* Volume 2, (1). 10.1037/tmb0000030

Elias, N. (1994). The *Civilizing Process.* Wiley & Sons, New York.

Goldhahn, E. (2007). *Shared habitats: the MoverWitness paradigm* [Doctoral Dissertation, Plymouth University].

Goldhahn, E. (2011). Being seen digitally: a filmic visualization of a "Long Circle". movers and witnesses in "Authentic Movement". In Birringer, J. and Fenger J. (Eds.), *Dance & choreomania* (pp. 248–258). Gesellschaft für Tanzforschung und Henschel Verlag.

Goldhahn, E. (2015). Towards a new ontology and name for Authentic Movement, *Journal of Dance and Somatic Practices,* Volume 7, 2, (pp. 273–285).

Goldhahn, E. (2017). *Long circle—so we are here now: three Authentic Movement films.* Films Media Group, USA, available online (last visited 13 July 2020).

Isaacs Russell, G. (2015). *Screen relations: the limits of computer-mediated psychoanalysis and psychotherapy.* Karnac Books.

Randow, v. G. (2020). Demokratie in zeiten des coronavirus, die biopolitische krise, *Die Zeit* (Issue 5th April 2020).

Chapter 12

The MoverWitness and science: an ecological turn

Introduction

This chapter was first published as an essay titled "Authentic Movement and Science" in *A Moving Journal* (2003), now no longer available online. Written prior to my formal arts-led research it appears in the context of this volume prompted by the singular urgency of our time: the climate crisis. The essay has been edited since its first publication and now uses the term MoverWitness (Goldhahn 2007, 2009a, 2015).

Twenty years ago my longing to connect creative embodiment and empathetic witnessing practices as a method with natural sciences was met and supported by the late Brian Goodwin, biologist and course convener at Schumacher College at Dartington, UK. Inviting me to teach BSc students of biology and holistic science, we aimed to introduce scientists to an awareness of their own bodies in movement and observation and to enable them to use this as a springboard to self-reflect within their science projects.

Holistic science as taught and researched at Schumacher College at that time is founded in the belief that all environments and habitats are shared between a multitude of factors and beings that need to be considered together rather than singled out. This view has been adopted in holistic science (Goodwin 1994, 2003; Bortoft 1996; Holdrege 1996; Thoma 2003; Wemelsfelder 2003).

Authentic Movement and Science (edited version 2021)

In observation of nature, large and small, I have constantly asked myself the question: Is this the object or is it myself, that speaks here?

(Goethe 1999, p. 40)

Originally written over 200 years ago, this aphorism by the German poet, philosopher and scientist Johann Wolfgang Goethe is poignant and timely today. The question of the observer's influence on the observed has raised questions over the past century in all the sciences. While the social sciences

DOI: 10.4324/9781003222309-16

have developed research on a qualitative basis, the natural sciences have less developed tools to track and chart complexities of interrelationship between observer and observed. A Cartesian scientific world view has dominated our understanding of earth and its beings and workings to the detriment we are facing now in the 21st century. A less known branch of science, holistic science, has quietly raised concerns but was long overheard. Holistic science incorporates the scientist's influence on her observation, it considers the object of research to be part of a whole.

Within MoverWitness practices the relationship between the observer and the observed is central to enquiry. Through my work with postgraduate scientists and biologists, I have come to think that it can provide a practical method for use by scientists to become more conscious and reflective of uncharted territories, namely their own bodily knowledge, their imagination, their intuition and their creativity as located and sourced from within themselves. Further I have come to believe that embodied observation combined with using detailed phenomenological percept language enables an empathetic and intellectual grasp of the inherent connections between a scientist and her 'subject'. In 2000, I had the opportunity to explore these ideas at Schumacher College in Devon, UK where I taught a 12-week course introducing MoverWitness within the context of holistic natural science. With one of my students, Heather Thoma, a continued, albeit geographically distant dialogue and mini-research project ensued, she in Canada and myself in Germany. (I had relocated in order to take up a full-time position as dance movement psychotherapist at a clinic for children and adolescents in Germany.) Our mini-research project culminated in a collaborative presentation at the Festival of the Arts, Sciences and Environment: Shared Habitat in Toronto in 2002.

For our collaborative project, we adopted each other's practices: hers, the practice of Goethean Science and mine, the MoverWitness. We hoped that for both of us, studying the other's discipline would reveal new aspects. In this article, I write about my emerging questions resulting from teaching creative dance and Authentic Movement to biologists and from collaborating with Thoma.

As a holistic approach to natural science, Goethean science endeavours to encompass the wholeness of an environment observed whilst taking account of the particularities of its details. But instead of dividing and singling out, as is common in reductionist science, Goethean science tries to understand the individual organism or phenomenon as a whole and within its surrounding context to which it is closely related. Goethe, who was critical of the evolving reductionist view, commented that theories are usually impatient results of a mind that wants to rid itself of the observable phenomena. It replaces these with images, terminology, even just words (Goethe 1999). Instead of theorising, Goethe adhered to phenomenological descriptions of what he witnessed in nature. He took time and was patient. He attuned with what he saw

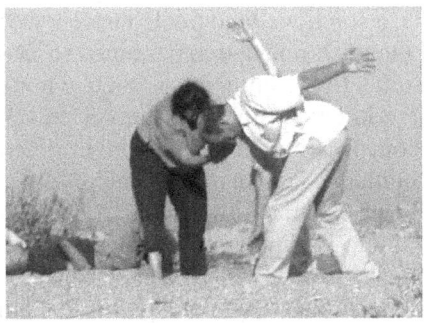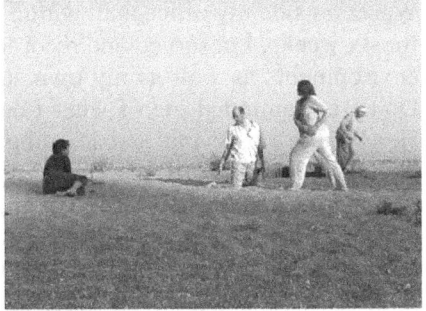

Figure 12.1 Slapton beach movers 1, two video stills. Artist: Eila Goldhahn, 2003

in nature. He was guided by his experiences of seeing and perceiving and reflected upon how these activities themselves provided him with new insights.

Goethe's method of observation is very similar to the practice of witnessing as I know and teach it in the MoverWitness. Learning about Goethean science from Thoma made me curious to understand and learn more about this way of practicing science. Until then, I had considered science to always inherently promote a Cartesian view of the world of creating perspective and claiming that this was the only one, of measuring, of weighing and of calculating, of creating absolute truths.

Expanding practice: the MoverWitness

Thoma and I engaged in each other's practice on a daily basis. Throughout the summer for 20 minutes daily, we observed a natural environment. Another 20 minutes, we engaged in contemplative movement practice, focusing on the development of inner witness qualities, such as holding an inner focus, being responsive to one's own emerging movement material, and, while moving, being aware of oneself. Each practice period was followed by writing in the first person and present time, a format that is used in percept language (see also Chapter 3 of this volume). Being in distant geographical locations, we agreed on coinciding in time and subsequently sharing our writing by e-mail. In this way we created a framework by which we increased the feeling of support and connectedness between us emphasising the inner nature and intentionality of the work.

Learning from each other we developed a four-step guide in observing natural environments near ourselves. The guide included tasks such as noting perceptions, preconceptions and fantasies, as well as using a contemplative, slow approach to observing an environment. I was working as a dance therapist at the time in Germany and chose a flood plain by the river Weser outside my office and, within this, a small wetland pool. Twice a week for six weeks, I observed and recorded the phenomena that pertained to these environments as well as my own self-reflective comments as their witness. Doing so reminded me of what I engage in as a witness to human movers. Here I was observing and learning about a complex natural environment, there I was observing and learning about the human body and psyche in its moving embodiment. In both, I was witnessing flow, movement, pattern, rhythm, shapes and stillness. In both, I found complexities and inter-relationships between different phenomena.

As in MoverWitness practice, I noticed that my perceptions became sharper and more alert and that increasingly my ability to remember details grew. I felt excited to note small changes and phenomena as I returned again and again to the same sites – there was a developing sense of knowing a place. Knowing the places made me also feel more at home: I experienced a growing inner attachment to the sites. This came about by disciplined regularity of my visits, by taking time to be in the sites and by consciously willing myself be in and with the sites.

Practising as a mover and a witness, I had over many years of practice developed an inner capacity to see myself and another. I had first developed my inner witness and then, resulting from that, a growing capacity to see others. I was using these skills in my practice of dance therapy. Adler (1987) describes certain developmental steps in the context of Authentic Movement as: 'I long to see another' and 'I see another'. These statements became relevant in my new environmental observations too. In my consider-ations of an environment, I found a strangely potent reflection of my own inner life, my moods, my feelings and even my projections, depending on what sort of a day I had in my practice with clients and colleagues or what else was going on in my life.

This made me wonder how and if scientists also experience this personal aspect in their work and how this could possibly affect or reflect in their work. Were scientists in a projective or an empathetic relationship with the environment or organism that they were studying? How would my own observations of environments be different if I had not practiced seeing and being seen by another? Would doing this work and being unaware of self-reflective processes or my own embodiment make a differ-ence to what I saw and how I noted it down? Would I see differently? Would I even remain unconnected where I felt a growing attachment? Might I see less?

As I am not a natural scientist the study of these natural phenomena engaged me, primarily, on a reflective, empathic and aesthetic level. I did not ask questions as to the how and why of what I saw. I did not investigate mechanisms or workings other than my method of attending, seeing, perceiv-ing and recording. Then understanding something new came in an entirely unexpected way. When observing plants in my sites I had found myself struck by their incredibly slow movement. Then, when I allowed myself to enter into the perceptual qualities of that slowness, I began to distinctly perceive the otherness and different life of the plant. I felt as though I had entered a different realm of being, one that was extremely slow and pertained to a different sense of time altogether. Whilst this otherness was striking in itself, almost simultaneously, I also became aware of another quality. This was a feeling of a new connectivity that seemed to tie me intimately to the plant. An entirely unexpected quality of equality emerged. I can liken this experience to my experience of being a witness to a mover, although I know that this sounds strange. Perhaps I felt empathy? At times, this new experience instilled a sudden and very urgent sense of respect for the individual plant or the small and complex environment that I observed. I sometimes felt as though a plant and I were coming face to face. At other times I felt as if a plant somehow grew larger within my perception than it actually was in my day-to-day view of it. I began to experience a very powerful sense of presence emanating from individual plants. All these new experiences shifted my perceptions away from me as being the active, powerful part to being somewhat down-sized in relationship to the plant. What I am describing here were not hallucinations or distortions of my perceptions but a new way of seeing and perceiving, one where my skill of witnessing allowed me into experiences of empathic attunement with a member of a different species. Perhaps this could be named as an interspecies-becoming?

Admittedly these experiences were awesome and bewildering. Adler's question Who is the witness? (Adler 1987) became my question of Who is the mover? As I felt to be the mover in the presence of a particular plant I was observing, a feeling arose from a deep and uncompromising part within myself, perhaps a part from childhood and of seeing things differently? Having always loved nature and working with the natural environment, gardening, planting trees, walking and swimming, this experience was new. It was also fleeting. I noticed how quickly a distraction would cause a shift in my perception. The experience (not the concept!) of deep respect for the plant as another being, one that somehow and unwittingly was witnessing me, would shift back to my normal state of perception and thinking, one in which I was 'superior'.

When I assessed this 'normality', it revealed itself as a relationship between me as the subject and the supposedly observed as an object with an unquestioned hierarchy being the connecting principle. On reflection, I found that my day-to-day experience and perception of myself in relationship to the natural world is founded upon these deeply embedded and difficult to track, presumably conditioned, assumptions. Alongside my observational experiences came the thought that what I was experiencing was perhaps closer to how things really were, except that acculturation had turned this deeper knowledge upside down. The backwards somersault in my perception opened an albeit small window into another, completely different view of reality, one of a palpable parity of beings.

Opening up perspectives

Do biologists in their often exclusive and long-term observation of a single species similarly attune to the temporal/spatial rhythm and differently scaled worlds of plants or animals? What is missed or added when attunement is or is not present in observation?

Modern reductionist science often involves the use of highly developed technical equipment, allowing for a very specific and narrow focus on the object of enquiry. Scientists can be seen to become extensions of these machines. Often rendered in static physical positions, their visual sense and intellectual processing capacity have become their foremost tools of knowing. Computer models replace immediate contact with the research object and provide instead a virtual aspect of reality. This method of choosing and valuing visual perceptions can exclude, ignore, or quickly dismiss other levels of possible responses: kinaesthetic, emotional and intuitive. The resulting, very particular aspects of reality that are observed can be processed and responded to by the intellect.

Through the practices of MoverWitness, the knowledge of one's perceptions and projections increases; the understanding of the observer's own viewpoint broadens. Bringing focus to an inner world of sensations, images and feelings one attains a reflective state, which in time allows one to become more mindful of both internal and external complexities of experience. This increased individual awareness is then practiced in the presence of others so that one develops a capacity to be present with oneself as well as in relation to others. By verbalising one's perceptions of self and others with careful phenomenological descriptions of different levels of perceptions, a complex and systemic understanding of reality can be experienced, one

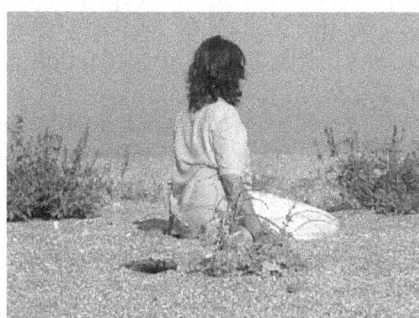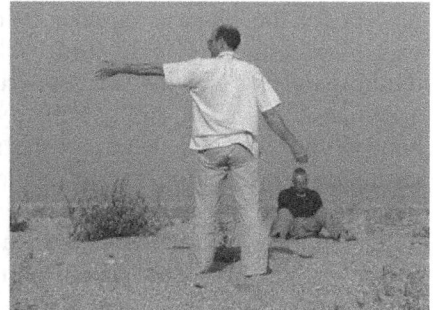

Figure 12.2 Slapton beach movers 2, two video stills. Artist: Eila Goldhahn, 2003

that can renew one's sense of perceptions to those which may have been available at a preverbal level of consciousness. Such perceptions can enrich intellectual enquiry.

First Slapton workshop

In response to my own observations, I designed a workshop around nature observation and elements of the MoverWitness for others, a mixed group of scientists and artists and for other student groups. Outcomes were participants' writing, verbal comments and a visual record, which I created by using camera-witnessing, as described in Chapters 3, 5 and 11 of this book.

I was present in the sessions as witness/facilitator, at times using the video camera. The presence of the video camera and the fact that we practiced MoverWitness in an outdoor environment made the set-up complex. Participants' safety and comfort were important to me and the group were extensively briefed as to what to expect. I had prepared a small instruction booklet with a number of experiential steps. The instructions given to the participants were based on elements from both the MoverWitness and Goethean Science, for example stating that

> Goethean Science is a way of looking at nature and observing it in a holistic way. Rather than the more common quantitative approach to science, one is looking at the qualities of a place and the relationships between the elements and creatures within it.

and that

> MoverWitness is a way of moving and being still, taking a contemplative look at one's inner world of sensations, feelings and images. Movement or stillness occurs from the inside out and one allows oneself to be seen by another in this process.

Participants' written responses

> I feel at one with my surroundings. I feel peaceful and sleepy. I can hear the wind and the waves. I can hear myself breathing and feel my heart beating for the first time today. The sun makes me think of summer, which makes me happy. (A., participant)

and

> I am lying on my front. The shingle is a mini-landscape, hills and valleys. Are they all from footprints? Or made by wind and rain?

Plastic litter trapped in the dry plant stalks – man! "Natural litter" of bits of wood and dead plants. The shingle is cold and appears sterile yet plants grow here and there, islands of growth. Always the sound of the sea, but I hardly notice its smell. Too cold for smells? I am watching to see if the shingle is moved by the wind - a piece of stalk moves across, noisily. People's footsteps on the gravel. I feel I don't want to move, as it will disturb the gravel. The gong sounds. (S., participant)

and

Warm sun, cool wind, wild irises – cat fish egg case – tingly sensation between toes of cold shingle [a pebbly beach] – note valerian shooting new green leaves out on beach. Distant ketch (or yawl) struggling to get out of Dartmouth Harbour. White spume from waves breaking on point to N.E. (D., participant)

The resulting short video provided a record in its own right, capturing the quality of the time and place, the movement and stillness, and the deep focus and contemplation that participants had entered into. Some participants seeing the video felt witnessed by its record. A growing awareness of the complexities involved made me plan other situations in which to explore these questions in more depth, both in the studio and out of doors. I continue to facilitate *Slapton beach mover* workshops and have created a number of short films about this ongoing arts and science project.

An ecological turn

Observations in holistic science and in the MoverWitness create relationships between seer and seen and dissolve subject–object relationships to a new parity, that of a mover and witness and vice versa. These relationships reveal complexities and the moment that is shared. In the moment of languaging, making a verbal statement about the observed, a new and conscious step of carefully holding the observed within the layer of communicable thought is required. The MoverWitness provides a practice that brings precision and clarity both to the originator of the perception, their thought and language, as well as to the other, the mover, the one who is made reference to. When honouring a phenomenology of perception knowledge, projections and imaginations of the scientist can become conscious.

It seems to me that the MoverWitness has much to offer the natural scientists, particularly today as scientists will have to deal with devastating observations of climate change. From developing greater capacities on perceptual levels to an awakening of creative intuition, to expanding awareness of projections, to the capacity for empathy for the environment and organism studied, and further to creating circles of support between humans and the natural environment: there are many avenues to be yet explored, all of which might help to provide us with the necessary ecological turn.

What matters most is that humans learn to no longer stand apart from nature. In a post-human and post-research world, formerly disparate disciplines are no longer as separate as once thought. To see ourselves and our makings, fabrications, machines, artificial intelligence, to be separate from nature reveals itself as being illusory in the face of ecological disaster, biosciences and the final realisation of the interconnectedness and dependency of all ecologies, things and organisms globally. The 2021 Nobel Prize in Medicine or Physiology was awarded to David Julius and Ardem Patapotian, from the US, who have been able to explain the profound workings of our proprioceptive interface with our way of knowing the world: touch, an inherent part of embodiment.

Almost 20 years after my initial experiments with MoverWitness and science a post-pandemic, climate-challenged world is calling for a fundamental shift in our ever more urgent reconciliation with nature. The role of scientists' embodiment, their relationship to their own bodies and its impact on their way of doing science was explored by Werner Kutschmann in *Der Naturwissenschaftler und sein Körper* (1986), a German book tracing the history of scientists' relationships with their bodies and in turn their way of doing science. A different way of thinking about nature has long been reflected upon by holistic scientists and thinkers Goodwin (1994, 2003), Abram (1996, 2021), Bush and Hoppe (1999), Heveker (1999), Pollan (2002), Todres (2002), Thoma (2003), Deleuze and Guattari (2004). In the field of embodiment and performance, there are many works that admonish and urge us, such as performative works by Annette Arlander *Meetings with Remarkable and Unremarkable Trees* (2021) and Miranda Whall (2021) who dresses up like a sheep to meet sheep in a literal becoming-animal, perhaps with a reference to Deleuze and Guattari's thinking. This is just citing a few individuals from the growing number of individuals and collaborators thinking and acting differently across all disciplines, arts and sciences.

The mystical writer Rofe (1960) stated that 'entering into the nature of a plant' may sound a strange idea to some. It is interesting to note how that which can no longer be considered rational science, has to fall within the realm of mysticism in order to be said at all. There are also earlier, astounding theories about a-causal relationships in observation of natural phenomena for example by Jung and physicist Ernst Pauli (1955). These ideas and observations touch upon intuitive embodiments mirrored in Plevin's exploration of quantum physics as a metaphor for chance encounters in Authentic Movement (Plevin 1999) and further related in terms of natural sciences in Goodwin (2003). There are many ways of sensing through movement and touching other beings around us in becoming tree, cow, sheep or seaweed and paying tribute to a belongingness of their predicament within a human-dominated world that is altering and destroying all shared habitats at this time on earth.

In the face of the repeated and increasingly severe droughts and heat-waves, we cannot but wonder about the effect of these events on the emotional and mental states of all beings but also on human scientists in particular. "Shocked climate scientists are wondering how even worst-case scenarios failed to predict such furnace-like conditions so far north" (Watts 2021). Further, Watts relates Johan Rockström (director of the Potsdam Institute for Climate Impact Research) stating that "the recent extreme weather anomalies were not represented in global computer models that are used to project how the world might change with more emissions. The fear is that weather systems might be more frequently blocked as a result of human emissions". Whilst eco-anxiety is a reasonable response, there is also widespread bewilderment and avoidance as "more people in more countries are feeling that their weather belongs to another part of the world". It must be time to change our way to perceive nature not as being separate from us, but as part and party to human and other-than-human life on this planet. Creative embodiment, empathy and a non-judgemental way to use language might help to support much needed peaceful collaborations between peoples and nations to ammeliorate the problems we have gotten ourselves into.

References

Abram, D. (1996). *Spell of the sensuous: perception and language in a more-than-human world*. First Vintage Books, New York.

Adler, J. (1987). Who is the witness, a description of Authentic Movement. *Contact Quarterly,* 12, no 1, 1987, (pp. 20–29).

Arlander, Anette (2021). *Meetings with Remarkable and Unremarkable Trees*. The International Center for Knowledge in the Arts, Denmark, Knowledge in the Arts #2. (March 30, 2021) [www.meetingwithtrees.com].

Bortoft, H. (1996). *The Wholeness of Nature: Goethe's Way of Science*. Lindisfarne Press, US.

Deleuze, G. & Guattari, F. (2004). Becoming-animal. Atterton, P. & Calarco, M. (eds.) Animal Philosophy (pp. 85–100). Continuum, London, New York.

Goethe, J. W. (1999). *Schriften zur Naturwissenschaft*. Edition Reclam.

Goldhahn, E. (2007). *Shared habitats, the MoverWitness paradigm*. [Doctoral dissertation, Dartington College of Arts and University of Plymouth, UK]

Goldhahn, E. (2009a). Is *authentica* meaningful name for the practice of Authentic Movement? *American Journal of Dance Therapy*. Volume 31, Issue 1, (p. 53–63).

Goldhahn, E. (2015). Towards a new name and ontology for the Discipline of Authentic Movement. *Journal of Dance and Somatic Practices,* 7: 2, (pp. 273–285).

Goodwin, B. (1994). *How the leopard changed its spots: the evolution of complexity*. Phoenix, London.

Goodwin, B. (2003). Patterns of wholeness: holistic science. *Resurgence, Patterns of wholeness,* Jan/Feb 2003, No. 216 (pp. 12–14).

Heveker, N. (1999). Formgebende Prozesse in der Biologie -Thema und Variation-. In *Bornstedter Dialoge: Farbe, Form, Kommunikation, Dynamische Prozesse in lebendigen Systemen,* Siegward Sprotte Stiftung Potsdam, Breklumer Verlag.

Holdrege, C. (1996). *Genetics and the manipulation of life.* Lindisfarne Press, US.

Hoppe E-G & Bush, A (1999) Die Sprache der Zellen. In *Bornstedter Dialoge: Farbe, Form, Kommunikation, Dynamische Prozesse in lebendigen Systemen,* Siegward Sprotte Stiftung Potsdam, Breklumer Verlag.

Jung, C. G. & Pauli, W. (1955). Synchronicity: a causal connecting principle. In *The Influence of Archetypal Ideas on the Scientific Theories of Kepler.* Routledge & Kegan Paul Ltd.

Kutschman, W. (1986). *Der Naturwissenschaftler und sein Körper: die Rolle der 'inneren Natur' in der experimentellen Naturwissenschaft der frühen Neuzeit.* Frankfurt. Suhrkamp.

Plevin, M. (1999). The movement of all things, Authentic Movement and quantum physics. *A Moving Journal* (1999), Volume 6, no. 2, (pp. 4–9).

Pollan, M. (2002). *The botany of desire: a plant's-eye view of the world.* Bloomsbury Publishing, London.

Rofe, H. (1960). *Reflections on Subud.* Humanity Publishing Company. Rogge, Amsterdam.

Shared Habitat 2: *Dance and biology, Festival of art, science and environment.* Conference proceedings, York, Toronto, 2003.

Thoma, H. (2003). All at the same time. *Resurgence, Patterns of wholeness,* Jan/Feb 2003, No. 216 (pp. 15–17).

Todres, L. (2002). Humanising forces: phenomenology in science; psychotherapy in technological culture. *The Indo-Pacific Journal of Phenomenology,* Volume 2, Edition 1, 4/2002, (pp. 1–11).

Watts, J. (2021). Canadian inferno: northern heat exceeds worst-case climate models: scientists fear heat domes in North America and Siberia indicate a new dimension to the global crisis. (2 July 2021). *The Guardian,* London. https://www.theguardian.com/environment/2021/jul/02/canadian-inferno-northern-heat-exceeds-worst-case-climate-models [last visited 4 October 2021].

Whall, M. (2021). www.mirandawhall.space [last visited 7 May 2021]

Postscript

Reflections on Authentic Movement has described, clarified and critiqued certain aspects of these practices. It has also suggested ways in which its knowledges might be shared and ways of practicing improved. It has explored connections with other disciplines (than therapy and mysticism) that I hope will benefit from its elegant workings. The numinous and the transpersonal have not been the focus of my writing in this volume; however, as I close, it is time to pay my respects. I have experienced such precious moments and know that they can occur wherever we may find ourselves, in and out of MoverWitness.

A few years ago, together with my cousin Martina, I visited the small German town of Kevelaer, a place of pilgrimage near the Dutch border. I had never heard of this town until my cousin mentioned it and suggested we visit as my husband was in search of a Madonna figure. The town had been founded on the premise of a mystical experience in 1641 by Hendrik Busman and a small chapel had been built around the site of this, with the town and a large cathedral having been built nearby. There were queues of people waiting to enter the chapel. When it was my turn, I stepped into the twilight gingerly approaching the holy site. My surprising experience was this: when I approached and stood still, I could not see what was in front of me, but I had the overwhelming sense that it was I who was seen instead.

Index